# 6 LIFE CHANGING ENERGY HEALING METHODS

## How to Release Emotional Stress, Pain and Illness

John O'Dwyer

Copyright © 2018 John O'Dwyer

All rights reserved.

Published by: Chi Choices, LLC
www.ChiChoices.com

ISBN: 978-0-9987904-0-4

# Contents

| | |
|---|---|
| Disclaimer | 1 |
| Why You Need to Read This Book | 3 |
| Introduction | 13 |
| Part I - Stress & Trauma | 21 |
| Chapter One - Emotional Stress Sabotages Health | 23 |
| Chapter Two - Trauma Triggers Disease | 31 |
| Part II - Energy Healing Tools & Concepts | 39 |
| Chapter Three - The Body and Energy | 41 |
| Chapter Four - Sensing Energy | 53 |
| Chapter Five - Energy Healing | 61 |
| Part III - Energy Healing Solutions | 73 |
| Chapter Six - Perform Emotional Acupuncture Without Needles | 75 |
| Chapter Seven - Expel an Emotion with a Refrigerator Magnet | 97 |
| Chapter Eight - Point Your Fingers at Your Face to Heal | 117 |
| Chapter Nine - Read and Repair the Body's Light | 131 |
| Chapter Ten - Use a Little Known System of the Body to Heal | 143 |
| Chapter Eleven - Oxygenate Your Blood in Minutes Lying Down | 155 |
| Final Thoughts | 169 |
| Appendix A: Resources | 173 |

# Disclaimer

The author of this book is *not* a doctor and nothing in this book should be taken *in any way* whatsoever as medical advice. Readers of this book need to consult with their doctors and health care professionals for *all* their medical needs and advice.

This book is written for *educational purposes* only—to make readers aware of some unique and little known methods of bringing body, mind, spirit and emotions into greater balance. When the body is better balanced, healing is easier, according to ancient man and many modern doctors agree.

Furthermore, all stories of energy balancing and stress reducing methods herein are unique. Should the reader employ any of the methods or equipment described in this book, the reader will most likely experience *different* results from those in this book. The reader could also have no results or even negative effects.

# Why You Need To Read This Book

We're living in a stressful world and this book will tell you how to deal with the terrible twins—stress and trauma—which cause us pain, make us sick and even kill us. They can deprive us of oxygen and wipe out our immune system.

So, what can you do? To start with, read this book. It's all about resolving various emotional and energetic stresses—often permanently. The result is less pain, discomfort and illness.

Most of the time, when I meet someone in intense physical or emotional pain, I can help them reduce that pain, using no equipment, within minutes. I do that by using just one method in this book which I've been using for well over a decade. This has happened so often that I am no longer amazed.

How did I learn about health? Well, at age 27, I took some food supplements, felt better, became a *health nut* and began researching health.

Since then, I've read hundreds of health books, yet I was definitely not immune myself from pain and stress, as you'll soon learn. But what I've learned may help you immensely.

It has already helped my mother, who turned 101

years young in mid-2016. She has used, and still uses, some of the energy healing methods in this book.

You may be needlessly suffering and feel you have no good health options. That was my situation for much of my life. Sports and exercise helped immensely in the short term, but they did not permanently remove my emotional stress.

If you have stress, discomfort or illness in your life, this book will give you some brand new, user friendly solutions with which most medical personnel are unfamiliar. Since most physicians don't personally use them, how could they recommend them to patients like yourself?

Here are a few simple questions. If you answer yes to any of them, then this book was written just for you.

1. Are you experiencing chronic aches, pain or discomfort?

2. Do you have a degenerative illness or an autoimmune disease?

3. Do you suffer from stress, trauma or emotional baggage?

4. Do you want to help a friend or loved one who has any of the above issues?

Many people, despite trying numerous medical procedures, remain in pain. They are told that drugs or surgery are the only solutions and that they are facing disability if they do nothing. Some doctors, to their credit, suggest exercise, meditation, recreation and vacation to help deal with stress.

We're all free to make our own health choices and my personal option is to avoid drugs which all have side effects. Even though my grandfather was a surgeon in Ireland, I believe surgery, while sometimes necessary, is rarely the answer to chronic aches and pain.

Doctors concentrate on treating *symptoms*, like tumors, instead of zeroing in on the *causes* of illness, which are often stress and trauma. Moreover, most doctors don't know how to eliminate stress and trauma.

**My Own Stress & Trauma**

My own life has seen excruciating pain, chronic stress and different types of trauma despite growing up in a small town in a loving and nurturing home environment. Here are a few of my stressful experiences:

1. In sixth grade, I fell off a wall head first onto a concrete sidewalk while playing hide and seek at night.

2. In junior high school, while roller skating, I fell and broke two front teeth and had a silver cap on one of them during all of my high school years.

3. Playing rugby, I suffered a concussion resulting

in a total loss of memory. I didn't even know my name, but fortunately all memory prior to the head blow returned within several hours.

4. My second rugby concussion was a few years later and my third concussion happened while snow skiing.

5. While attending the United States Naval Academy, I was in a state of chronic stress during the first year, called Plebe Year. Most nights I just wanted to go to bed and not wake up, due to being subjected constantly to the stress of *character building,* which some call hazing. Despite it all, I did graduate.

6. When I was 19 years old, my father died unexpectedly at age 58 from a cerebral hemorrhage.

7. President Kennedy was assassinated on one of my birthdays.

8. While fast asleep in the middle of the night on a submerged nuclear submarine in the Pacific Ocean, I heard the announcement, "Flooding in the engine room." It was just a minor leak. Otherwise, you might not be reading these words.

9. Low back problems plagued me during five decades, despite treatment by chiropractors in California, Tokyo, Montreal and Mississippi.

10. In 2005, while we were hiding out in Florida, Hurricane Katrina destroyed one exterior wall of our Mississippi home, allowing intense winds and water from the Gulf of Mexico to enter our house and destroy much of its interior. We lost most of what we owned, including several automobiles. My mother's home was also flooded and she lost a car.

You undoubtedly have your own lengthy list of stressful and traumatic experiences which come with living on planet earth.

## Back Pain Problems

About 1980, while working in Japan, I experienced low backache which had bothered me, off and on, for over a decade. One night, I woke up screaming, unable to find any position in which there was no sciatic nerve pain. In the morning, bent over sideways, I took the train with my wife and saw an orthopedic doctor at the naval base in Yokosuka.

He told me to take several months off work, do nothing, and let my back heal. If I could not do that, he recommended surgery—something alien to my health philosophy. For a second opinion, he put me in touch with an English speaking Japanese neurosurgeon in Yokohama who simply said, "It's not cancer."

Then and there, I decided to live with it. Warmer weather helped it heal. Tennis, even in nice weather, usually resulted in severe low back pain so I gave it up

—for 30 years—until after I'd discovered some of the healing techniques in this book.

My Japanese chiropractor in Tokyo suggested that gentle running might be beneficial for my back. I tried a little jogging, something I loved doing for much of my life. However, the streets in my Japanese neighborhood were heavily sloped toward the gutter making it impossible to run evenly so I stopped.

Back in the United States, I told an American chiropractor in California that my Japanese chiropractor had told me gentle running would help my back. He said, "It's bad for the back" and stated he'd fix my back in a month or two.

After several months of unsuccessful chiropractic treatments with him, I cautiously started jogging on dirt and grass with new shoes, running for only a few minutes. I slowly increased my distances, joined a running club, and ran with the slowest runners. After I finished a half marathon six months later, my chiropractor repeated, "It's bad for the back."

Six months later, I completed a full marathon, 26 miles and 385 yards in 4 hours and 13 minutes—with no back problems. My chiropractor again stated, "It's bad for the back." I seldom, if ever, visited him again.

Fast forward about a quarter of a century. Using EFT, one of the healing techniques we'll cover in Part III of this book, I'm able to resolve most of my back and other pain issues by myself—in minutes—instead of days or weeks.

**Voice Victim**

Around the year 2000, I'd go to work, talk for half an hour or so, then sometimes be hoarse for the rest of the day. This was devastating as I love to talk and had been a lector in church for a quarter of a century. This condition persisted, off and on, for a year or two.

My wife suggested I contact a lady voice therapist who attended our church. I did that and she put me in touch with a nearby voice clinic. There they put a tube down my throat, videotaped my vocal cords and discovered an enormous hemorrhaged polyp on one vocal cord.

They gave me two options: anti-reflux drugs or surgery. I refused both, telling them I would find a way to correct it myself.

Despite being a health nut for around 30 years, I had no idea how to proceed, so my first resort was to prayer, a worldwide form of energy healing, which resulted in immediate results—within an hour—inside a second hand store.

Looking around that store, my good fortune there was to find and buy a number of used audio tapes about acidity, alkalinity, coral calcium and related subjects with which I was unfamiliar. Listening to them, I learned that disease cannot exist in a sufficiently alkaline body.

Within days, I began taking alkaline coral calcium, a product sold in the world's first drugstore in Madrid, Spain. My lunch was often an alkalizing salad. I monitored my urine pH multiple times a day and pursued an alkalizing diet since I then knew that the cells of the body work best when slightly alkaline.

After maybe 2–3 months, the polyp was already smaller. They were all amazed at the voice clinic as they'd never seen such a dramatic improvement as mine and we had photos to prove it. The polyp shrank so fast that I later created a website giving some information about acidity, alkalinity, oxygen and more. My website is:

www.ChiChoices.com.

Unfortunately, my polyp photos, which I planned to share later with others, were lost in Hurricane Katrina.

I understand pain and know how helpless it feels to be without the knowledge of the many energy healing options presented in this book—*none* of which I knew about when I was simply alkalizing my body. Curiously enough, reducing stress makes the body more alkaline, allowing it to function better and heal more rapidly.

While there exist *many* effective ways to heal the body which are not in this book, I have chosen to include only those which my wife and I have used. Moreover, I have been awarded certificates in several of them and have used them to help many individuals.

In my *Introduction*, you'll see why this book is different from any one you have yet to read.

# Introduction

As you've read, I'm a long time health nut. Over 4–5 decades I have slowly accumulated information unknown to most Western doctors.

Western doctors believe that stress and trauma contribute to pain, discomfort and illness. But, unfortunately, they're largely unaware of the *numerous* ways to eliminate stress and trauma, some of which are detailed in this book.

My search for better health has led me to accumulate knowledge of many energy healing modalities that I want to share with you in this book.

**Personal Health Research**

Since 1971, I've read hundreds of books on nutrition, alternative health, energy healing and other health topics. Even though I lost some 200 health books in Hurricane Katrina, I've read many others since.

Most of the books I've read this century aren't in your local library as they are very unusual and little known. Your physician has probably not read most of them.

In the early 1970s, I attended several medical conferences. At one of those, the speaker was one of the famous Canadian Shute brother doctors. At that time these doctors had successfully treated many thousands of Canadians with vitamin E for heart issues.

About that time, the United States had *no* minimum daily requirement for vitamin E, even though much of the world knew it was extremely beneficial to health in many different ways.

Some veterinarians were ahead of our medical doctors. Those vets had a racehorse named Secretariat running on vitamin E. In 1973, that horse won the famous Triple Crown—the first horse to do so in 25 years.

My health research has spanned many decades. You may have neither the time nor inclination to investigate health, so I feel compelled to share my knowledge with you. It is my way of giving back to others.

So what have I done? I have used many different medical methodologies, including: electrodermal screening, cold lasers, energy machines, Dr. Navarro's HCG urine test for cancer, homeopathy, iridology, essential oils and many energy healing methods that will be explained in this book. My family, including my 100+ year old mother drink hexagonal alkaline water. I seek holistic health approaches to various ailments of the body.

I go to biologic dentists, make my own colloidal silver, do coconut oil pulling and think highly of alternative medical treatments, some of which have been around for millennia. I put no pharmaceutical medication into my body. The last aspirin I took was sometime in

*Introduction*

the 1960s.

## Reversing Health Problems

In this book I will introduce you to these people who turned to energy healing to reverse pain, stress and illness:

1. A disabled man in constant pain who used The Emotional Freedom Techniques (EFT) to reverse his multiple sclerosis, start his own business and become independent again.

2. A 4-year-old boy who started talking in complete sentences the day after several stuck emotions were dislodged using The Emotion Code.

3. A medical doctor whose *incurable* ALS (Lou Gehrig's Disease) disappeared after using Healing Codes for about 3 months. He just said some words and pointed his fingers at his face and neck a number of times a day in special sequences.

4. A horse owner whose horse was able to conceive after it had received two Biophoton Therapy treatments.

5. An Olympic diver who eventually solved her vertigo problem—and other medical issues—by turning to Craniosacral Therapy (CST) after trying numerous treatments without success.

6. A lady who had lost the use of one and a half lungs who used the Original Chi Machine to regain full use of both lungs. It also reversed her congestive heart failure and healed her brain after a tumor was removed.

We instinctively know that excessive stress is detrimental to our health. Doctors also know this so they often encourage their patients to avoid or minimize stress. Stress is often brought under control when we are relaxing, listening to music, practicing *tai chi* or meditating.

This book is primarily focused on eliminating many *sources* of our stress, pain, trauma or chronic disease. Some of the methods in this book can correct faulty thinking and even *permanently* release stresses and traumas behind our discomfort and illnesses.

In my opinion and that of an ever growing number of doctors, the methods in this book are vastly superior to *talk therapy* in releasing stress, trauma and emotional baggage lurking behind chronic illness. Modern energy healing methods often work quickly without having to dredge up old hurts during therapy.

These techniques are relatively new, with several of them being developed or just becoming more popular within the past decade or two. They are largely unknown to doctors as they are usually not taught in medical schools. Unfortunately, most doctors cannot eliminate the stress and trauma behind discomfort and illness.

*Introduction*

While I'm not a doctor, nor desire to be, I do hold certificates in several energy balancing techniques. I've gotten hundreds of individuals pain free, or largely free of physical pain or emotional stress in minutes using just one of them—with no equipment.

Furthermore, I have conducted hundreds of sessions using another technique which is discussed in this book. My wife and I have also paid certified practitioners to work on us using the healing arts described in this book.

The body heals itself whenever the immune system is working properly. Stress and trauma compromise our immune function, making it very difficult for us to fight illness. This book is about reducing—or completely eliminating—stress, trauma and emotional baggage.

**My Love of Energy Healing**

This book is about healing with energy and I possess certifications in these energy balancing modalities:

1. The Emotional Freedom Techniques (EFT); and

2. The Emotion Code; and

3. The Body Code.

My wife and I have used all of them in addition to Quantum Neuro Reset Technique (QNRT), The Healing Code, Three Dimensional Therapy (T3),

Biophoton Therapy, Craniosacral Therapy and others, including the Original Chi Machine and other energy machines.

Energy healing is wonderful for humans and I will relate many examples of that. Since some energy healing methods can also be used with your pets, I'll also share some interesting stories about healing animals.

**What This Book Covers**

**Part I: Stress & Trauma.** This section reveals how emotional stress and trauma, lodged in the body, compromise our health, causing discomfort and disease. Trauma and stress are enemies of the immune system and they must be controlled or, ideally, eradicated for us to truly recover from pain, discomfort and disease.

There are many stressors within the body. This book concentrates on dealing with emotional stress and trauma which are hard for doctors to diagnose, control or eliminate. However, they must be dealt with because they undermine good health.

**Part II: Energy Healing Tools & Concepts.** In this part, we will discuss energy and some tools which can be used in energy healing. You will learn about *muscle testing* and how it can be used to interrogate the subconscious mind and get *yes* and *no* answers to your questions.

Other topics are *intuition, energetic healing, healing*

*at a distance* and *intention*. These are used by various energy healing techniques in Part III of this book.

**Part III: Energy Healing Solutions.** Six unique ways to heal yourself—and possibly your pets—with energy are described. You can perform some of these yourself and others can be done with a practitioner, even *long distance* with someone in another state or country. The average doctor is probably not familiar with any of these.

Your ultimate mission—if you decide to accept it—is to consider using one or more of these energy healing methods. You might just lose some or all of your pain, trauma, emotional baggage, or illnesses, leading to improved health and inner peace.

# Part I

# STRESS & TRAUMA

# Chapter One

## EMOTIONAL STRESS SABOTAGES HEALTH

Emotional stress is caused when we do not have positive coping methods to deal with stressful situations in our life—which can be anything from sitting in traffic, to interacting with our boss, co-workers or family members, to dealing with financial pressures and medical issues.

Emotional stress is detrimental to health because, when stress is not dealt with properly, it gets stored in our cells, tissues and organs. This stored stress will often result in irritation, inflammation, discomfort, pain and illness.

It can also throw us into what's called the *fight or flight* state. This mode makes our cells more acidic, deprives us of oxygen, negatively impacts our immune system, and makes us prone to disease.

Let's look at the effects of stress on our health.

**Stress Gets Stored in Our Body**

When we don't handle the emotions related to stress

properly, those negative emotions can get trapped in the tissues of our body and impact our organs and overall health. Emotional stresses can originate at any time during our lives, including when we are in the womb.

Like genes, emotions can be inherited from our parents. We'll learn much more about that later in Part III where emotions are treated in considerable detail.

The ancient Chinese believed that emotions were created by various organs of the body. Certain emotions have been traditionally linked with specific paired organs, one a *yin* organ and the other a *yang* organ. Fear is linked with the kidneys or bladder, anger with the liver or gallbladder and grief with the lung or colon.

Let's say we're at a shopping mall and spot an ideal parking place, but another person steals *our* spot—the one we were waiting for. The anger we feel is created by the liver or gallbladder. If we have a positive way to cope with this, perhaps by saying a prayer or using compassion to try to understand the other person's actions, we can process the anger and it will dissipate.

But if we don't deal with the anger properly, then the negative emotional energy of anger is stored *inside* the body. Each unprocessed emotion is stored in just one location.

Eric Robins, MD, contributing author to *The Heart of Healing* book, says the anger usually ends up in the smooth muscles of the body, perhaps in a knee, hip or

## Emotional Stress Sabotages Health

lung—but it can be stored anywhere. The location is often a weaker part of the body, perhaps due to an injury or illness.

These stored emotions irritate surrounding tissues, affect the flow of energy within the body, then may cause us irritation, inflammation, discomfort, pain and illness. This can happen quickly—or years later.

If emotional energy such as anger or frustration gets stuck in a lung, it can contribute to breathing problems, lung cancer and other lung problems later in life. Similarly, emotional energy stuck in the heart may lead to heart palpitations, heart attacks and other heart problems.

A common understanding in energy healing is that *the issues are in the tissues*. Massage therapists report that clients sometimes experience deep emotions during a massage.

Emotions are energy and, when the tissue holding the emotion is massaged, the client may feel the emotion being *activated*, which can leave the client in tears or overwhelmed with deep feelings. This is evidence that our bodies harbor emotions and lock them in our tissues when we don't handle our emotions in a healthy way.

There are also interesting stories of organ recipients experiencing emotions from their organ donor. Again, this shows how emotions can reside in our organs, tissues and cells.

## Stress Depletes Oxygen from Our Cells

Without oxygen, we face brain damage and then death —in minutes. Because stress is so potent, it interferes with the oxygen in our bodies in numerous ways.

Oxygen is the cornerstone of healthy cells. In fact, cells deprived of sufficient oxygen can become cancerous. This was discovered by a little known medical doctor and biochemist, Otto Warburg, MD and PhD.

He studied the interaction between cellular oxygen and cancer and received a Nobel Prize in 1931 for proving, among other things, that:

1. *lack of oxygen* in our cells is the *cause* of cancer; and

2. that *oxygen kills cancer cells.*

His research illustrates how important oxygen is to healthy cell function because low oxygen can initiate cancer. He connected oxygen deficits with acidic cells because insufficient oxygen inside the body results in acidic cells.

Acidity and alkalinity are measured by pH, short for *potential of hydrogen*. The pH scale ranges from 0, the most acidic, to 14, the most alkaline. A pH below 7 indicates acidity and above 7 indicates alkalinity. A pH of 7 is neutral, neither acidic nor alkaline. A healthy cell should have a pH of 7.365, slightly alkaline.

Most of the cells inside the body should be alkaline, apart from the stomach and parts of the digestive tract which are acidic when digesting food. The skin, on the other hand, should always be acidic.

Unfortunately, emotional stress makes us *very* acidic inside, depriving us of oxygen, as we'll now see.

## Stress Puts Us in Fight or Flight Mode

Most of the time, we are in the *rest and digest* mode. It allows us to fight off disease, digest food and operate normally.

Dr. Walter Cannon, a Harvard physiologist, coined the name *fight or flight* in the early 1900s to describe what happens when the lives of mammals are in mortal danger.

Hans Selye, MD, PhD, known as the *Father of Stress,* conducted experiments decades later linking stress with disease. At the University of Montreal, starting in 1936, he became the world's expert on stress over many decades. He was nominated several times for the Nobel Prize for his research on stress.

Dr. Selye determined that stress affects *every* member of the body which is why stress is linked to all illnesses. He authored many books. In one of them, *The Stress of Life,* he wrote:

> We have learned that stress is an inherent element of all disease.

Emotional stress becomes detrimental to our health whenever we go into the *fight or flight* mode. Once in a while is normal when we have to deal with a real crisis.

Let's say a bear is chasing us. When our brain recognizes this threat, we automatically go into the *fight or flight* mode. The *hypothalamus* in the brain sends a signal to the master gland, the *pituitary gland* at the base of the brain. The pituitary gland then signals the *adrenal glands,* located above our kidneys, to release adrenaline, cortisol and other acidic hormones into the bloodstream.

One purpose of this flood of hormones is to give us maximum muscle strength so we can better fight or flee the bear. But these hormones make our bodies very acidic. Acidic fluids mean less available oxygen which, as we learned above, can lead to cancer.

*Fight or flight* also causes the immune system to shut down so that we can direct all of our energy to fight or flee. But when the immune system is shut down, it is no longer able to protect us from pathogens and disease.

The digestive system also shuts down so that enormous amount of energy normally used for digesting food can be diverted to the current crisis. Poor digestion gives rise to many health problems due to not extracting essential nutrients from our food.

The *fight or flight* mode is supposed to serve us when we are under extreme duress—to push our body into high alert to save our life. But these situations are

## Emotional Stress Sabotages Health

usually *not* life and death situations. Instead, they are emotionally stressful situations involving our boss, children, finances, relationships, drivers and other people.

So, *fight or flight* becomes the default mode for dealing with most of life's emotional stresses. Unfortunately, this puts excessive strain on the body. If we experience new stresses—or even just *think* about past emotionally stressful situations—the following important systems are shut down much of the time:

1. our immune system which heals the body; and

2. our digestive system which nurtures the body.

The increased acid from stress in our bloodstream decreases available cellular oxygen—a condition hazardous to our health. We don't need that acidity. Dr. Theodore Baroody, in his book *Alkalize or Die,* mentions that *all* the methods of natural healing he has investigated make the body more alkaline in the long run.

Getting rid of emotional stress and baggage makes us more alkaline and gives us more oxygen. Fortunately, there are many energy healing means to permanently release emotional stress and/or boost oxygen in the body. We'll walk through a number of them in Part III of this book.

# Chapter Two

## TRAUMA TRIGGERS DISEASE

We've discussed emotional stress which includes worry, tension, anxiety, fears, phobias, mental anguish and other kinds of emotional baggage.

Now let's look at trauma.

**What is Trauma?**

Trauma is a *sudden* and *intense* event. Trauma is *shock*. Trauma can occur whenever our life is in imminent danger—during a bank robbery, a terrorist attack or in wartime.

It can be *physical,* perhaps due to an automobile crash, a knife or bullet wound or resulting from a physical blow received in boxing, football or domestic violence. Sometimes physical trauma is so intense that, without quick action, the body may be unable to recover. For this reason, we have trauma centers.

Trauma can also be *mental* and *emotional* which occurs when someone threatens your life with a gun, after your loved one dies unexpectedly or upon learning you have a dreaded disease.

Even though we experience trauma, we rarely visit a trauma center. I already mentioned several personal traumatic experiences including 3 concussions, numerous falls, unexpected death, Hurricane Katrina and others.

I've also been laid off a number of times and that's why my family moved from California to Mississippi in early 1994. Before moving, I experienced one of the most traumatic events of my life.

I was in a deep sleep about 4:30 am when I was violently thrown up and down. I heard crashing in our house as books in a wall-to-wall bookcase were thrown everywhere. What went through my mind was, "This is the end of the world." I was mistaken.

It was the Northridge Earthquake, a rare one which moved the earth vertically instead of back and forth. Fearing aftershocks, we and our neighbors all went outside. Everyone experienced some trauma, especially my neighbor, Jim, who was still on his way home after working that night.

Jim was on the freeway when the quake occurred and he saw, in his rear view mirror, the freeway connector collapsing behind him and saw cars falling off the road to the ground far below. Had the earthquake hit seconds earlier, he would have plunged to his death. He arrived home shaking and traumatized.

Over a decade later, in 2005, many of my family and friends suffered *emotional* trauma in the aftermath of Hurricane Katrina. Other people, who chose to stay in their homes *during* Katrina, suffered *physical* trauma

—or even death.

Life can be traumatic and we are all affected by traumatic stress.

## Effects of Trauma

Individuals suffering from trauma may have anxiety, sadness, angry outbursts, poor concentration, troubled sleep, nightmares, panic attacks, depression, poor personal relationships, addictions, inability to move forward in life and other symptoms.

Thousands of veterans have Post Traumatic Stress Disorder (PTSD) as a result of the terrors and horrors of war. The methods in Part III of this book have quickly helped many veterans—even after no results during decades of medication and counseling.

When we have trouble coping with life, bad things—such as cancer—can happen within the body.

## Trauma and Cancer

Ryke Geerd Hamer, MD, was a medical doctor and cancer researcher in Germany. In 1978, his son was shot and died several months after that.

Dr. Hamer, who had always been very healthy, was diagnosed a few months later with testicular cancer, which he believed was triggered by the shock of his son's death. He decided to investigate further.

He examined the cancer patients he was following and discovered that *all* of them had experienced a traumatic shock somewhat prior to the onset of their cancer. He also discovered that each kind of trauma affects a particular part of the brain, which then affects some corresponding organ of the body.

He later determined that *all* diseases have an unexpected shock as a trigger. Some doctors today believe traumatic stress can initiate cancer—and other illnesses—from a few weeks to a year or two later.

Dr. Hamer developed a revolutionary way of treating disease which he called *German New Medicine*. It involves a radical way of looking at cellular health and healing. He developed *Five Biological Laws* and saw each disease as in either a *Conflict Active Phase* or in a *Healing Phase*.

Getting rid of the trauma allows us to better move into the Healing Phase where the body knows how to heal. So, one of the goals of Dr. Hamer and German New Medicine is to treat the trauma *behind* cancer or any illness

He treated or studied some 44,000 patients and healed many patients using his own unique methods. In addition to whatever medical procedures he used for cancer and other diseases, his treatment included *healing the traumatic shock* which had triggered the illness. By doing so, his results were incredible.

Some 6,000 of about 6,500 of his cancer patients, most deemed terminal, were free of cancer after 5 years. That is about a 92% success rate! Conventional medicine, at best, would reverse cancer in only a few percent of terminal cancer patients.

See the *Resources Appendix* for additional information on German New Medicine.

Be aware that a few of the methods in Part III of this book did *not* exist until very recently. According to some doctors, many of them have the potential to deal with traumatic stress even more quickly and effectively than those used by Dr. Hamer.

## The Shock Mode

In the last chapter, we learned we are in the normal slow *rest and digest* mode *or* in the fast *fight or flight* crisis mode. These are the only Western medicine neurological modes.

The ancient Chinese disagreed with modern medicine in many ways. For example, they had twice as many neurological modes. Here are their 4 modes, with names I've simplified:

1. **Relax mode.** This is the Western medicine *rest and digest* mode. We are calm and relaxed in this mode and the body can digest food.

2. **Alert mode.** This is the Western medicine *fight or flight* mode which gives us the strength we need during a crisis. Our ancestors may have been in this mode when confronted by a wild animal. Modern man may be in this mode when driving a car in heavy traffic.

3. **Sleep mode.** This is the mode designed for body repair and healing at night.

4. **Shock mode.** This mode is a type of *trauma* mode in which we tune out pain. People in this mode might walk on a broken leg while feeling no pain. Lives of people in this mode often hang in the balance. People in this mode may need trauma centers.

Medical schools used to teach that we are only in one mode at any given time. Nowadays, doctors are being taught that we can be, and usually are, in more than one mode at the same time. That's good, because whenever we are totally in the *fight or flight* high alert mode, our immune system is completely shut down.

According to acupuncturist Janice Walton-Hadlock, author of *Recovery From Parkinson's*, people with Parkinson's Disease of an unknown cause, called idiopathic Parkinson's Disease, are *all* in the *shock* mode which she calls the *dissociation* or *feel no pain* mode. They drift into and out of it throughout the day.

She found that most of these individuals had suffered a foot injury. When that happens, the stomach acupuncture meridian reverses. This situation is designed to be temporary—until the foot heals. But if we block the pain, then we may never heal and may be in the *shock* mode much of the time.

She has reversed so-called *incurable* Parkinson's Disease for many people, *including herself,* suffering from idiopathic, but not from drug-induced Parkinson's disease. The key was treating the foot problem with Chinese massage called *tui na* in conjunction with healing the stressful emotions behind the *shock* mode.

Many of her patients did *not* recover from Parkinson's Disease because they were unable to correct the stress and trauma keeping them, at least part of the time, in the *shock* mode. As I've mentioned, some of the energy healing methods in Part III of this book have the potential to greatly accelerate the healing of traumatic stress. In my opinion, they go far beyond the methods mentioned in her book.

We need a healthy balance between the *alert, relax* and *sleep* modes, as we are seldom totally in one mode or another. The *shock* mode is a trauma mode and is not a normal mode. We should rarely be in it and only for short periods of time.

## Healing Traumatic Stress

There are many methods of permanently ridding the body of stressful traumas. Most doctors are *not* familiar with any of them. On the other hand, my wife and I have used *all* 6 energy healing methods detailed in this book. My centenarian mother has used some of them—and still does.

Since trauma is energy, it is best removed with energetic healing methods, some of which are found in Part III of this book. You may wish to explore one or more of those methods further if you have trauma or disease in your life.

In Part II, we'll look at some principles of energy healing and some tools which are used by the energy healing methods described in Part III.

# Part II

# ENERGY HEALING TOOLS & CONCEPTS

# Chapter Three

## THE BODY AND ENERGY

The body has its own built-in wisdom and the ability to heal itself—provided the energy in the body allows it. Let's look at energy in the body and see how it correlates with health.

**What is Energy?**

The short answer is: everything.

Every substance is composed of energy—including living things like humans, animals and plants as well as non-living things like a table or chair. When we examine any material under a powerful microscope, we see that nothing is solid. Everything is made up of fields of energy which look like flies buzzing around.

Albert Einstein's famous formula $E=MC^2$ proved that matter and energy are interchangeable and that even a small amount of matter is equivalent to a large amount of energy.

Nuclear reactors make use of this as I well know since I've studied nuclear reactor physics and served as a nuclear trained submarine officer in the United States

Navy.

Bombs also convert matter to energy as I've known since the 1950s. Back then, in the car on my way to elementary school in Nevada, I witnessed the telltale *mushroom cloud* of an above ground atomic bomb blast conducted perhaps 100 miles away.

**Energy and Health**

For centuries, man has deemed overall health to involve that of:

1. the body
2. the mind
3. the spirit

Ancient man believed in balance of these three areas. When any one of these was out of balance, you were sick. When they were in harmony, you were well. This was the thinking of the Greeks and of other early civilizations we'll learn more about in this chapter.

The body is made up of trillions of cells. We've already seen how important cellular energy is. When oxygen is lacking, cancer and other illnesses often result.

One of my heroes is the late Dr. Emmanuel Cheraskin, a dentist, medical doctor and biochemist. He believed that we are only as healthy as our weakest individual cells, much like a chain is only as strong as its weakest link.

It is now well known that our cells are affected by the

mind, spirit and our emotional state. So, instead of concentrating solely on proper cellular nutrition—which is important—we also need to improve the quality of our mind, thoughts, spirit and emotions.

**Mind Power**

Our thoughts are energy and they deeply affect us. Abraham Lincoln once said, "Most folks are as happy as they make up their minds to be." Thoughts and words are powerful. Our own thinking can make us happy or unhappy. It can also make us sick or heal us. Our thinking not only affects *every* cell of our body but also impacts our genes.

If we think we'll get sick at age 80, 65 or 40, it usually happens, as our thoughts are somehow directing our cells to follow their wishes. This is called the *self-fulfilling prophesy*.

I recently told a young man in his 30s that my mom was 101 years old and he immediately said, "I don't think I'll live to be 100." I then gave him a quick explanation of the power of the mind.

Just believing that some new pill will help us can make it happen. This belief is so powerful that in clinical trials someone believing their pill was useful often got better—even if that pill contained *none* of the beneficial substance. This phenomenon is called the *placebo effect*.

Herbert Benson, MD, author of *The Relaxation Response* book, has long been interested in stress reduction techniques. Back in the 1980s, he traveled to Tibet to study the meditation of Tibetan monks.

Using meditation, the monks could stay warm when outside in the cold by increasing their skin temperature up to 17 degrees Fahrenheit. They could also wrap wet sheets around their bodies in 40 degree Fahrenheit temperatures and get the sheets so hot they gave off steam as they dried. Those monks impressed Dr. Benson with their mental prowess.

We'll discuss positive thinking and focused thoughts in another chapter. Meanwhile, let's look more at our minds.

**Our Two Minds**

Our mind has two components: the *conscious* mind and the *subconscious* mind. These two parts of our mind have been compared to an iceberg where the conscious mind is the 10–15% above the water and the subconscious mind is the 85–90% below the water.

When we use our conscious mind, we're aware of what we're saying and doing. However, we really don't know what's in our subconscious mind, although *muscle testing* and *intuition*, described in the next chapter, can help access it.

The subconscious mind functions like a computer running nonstop programs. These programs or habits are powerful. Some are helpful and others hurt us. So, if we want to change, we must alter our subconscious programming.

Our subconscious mind is a bully who wants to

control the often more passive conscious mind.

When we first learn to walk, ride a bicycle, drive a car, use chopsticks or exercise equipment, we do so consciously, thinking about each step. Over time, those motions learned with our conscious mind penetrate the subconscious mind and we no longer have to think about doing them. They become automatic.

Our two minds are connected. Thoughts start with the conscious mind and then, over time, they move into the subconscious mind and become part of our basic programming and habit database. So, if we want to make something automatic, we must alter our subconscious programs—often a challenging task.

## The Powerful Subconscious Mind

Habits and new beliefs are not created instantly because it takes time for information from the conscious mind to penetrate the subconscious mind. Experts believe it takes three weeks—or even much longer—to change our subconscious mind and form a new habit or way of thinking.

By repeatedly telling ourselves the same things, we brainwash ourselves and conscious thoughts eventually work their way into our subconscious mind. Giving suggestions to ourselves is called *autosuggestion.*

Our subconscious beliefs also change when we hear the same statements, over and over again, from parents and others. Once inside our subconscious mind, those beliefs become difficult to change. Some beliefs are beneficial, while others are toxic, adversely impacting our health.

The power of the subconscious mind was tragically demonstrated to me by three wonderful ladies I've known. Prior to being diagnosed with cancer, each of them was *adamantly* opposed to chemotherapy. One had had an earlier bad experience with conventional cancer therapies, another was training to become a naturopathic doctor and the third was skilled in the Japanese energy healing art of *reiki*.

They all, however, later underwent chemotherapy treatment and, unfortunately, each of them soon died. Although these individuals felt strongly that chemotherapy was not a beneficial treatment for their cancer, their subconscious programming was seemingly ok with chemotherapy.

Why was that?

Well, the subconscious mind is the bully and can overpower the passivity of the conscious mind when the two are not in sync. Perhaps my sick friends each had, even from childhood, one of these 4 subconscious beliefs:

1. always do what the doctor says

2. alternative medicine is risky

3. chemotherapy is mainstream

4. don't think outside the box

Those are just 4 possibilities. However, we all have thousands of beliefs and any number of them could conflict with our conscious desire with regard to medical treatment—or any other decision. Which ones affected my friends, I cannot say. But, I do know that the subconscious mind is extremely powerful.

Now let's move from mental energy to spiritual energy.

**Spiritual/Emotional Energy**

This is the energy of the *heart*, the energy of both positive and negative emotions. Improving emotional health is often considered part of spiritual healing, so I'll treat them together here.

Emotions are universally associated with the heart and spirit. When I was studying French in France, my professor once discussed the many French expressions containing the French word for *heart*. English is no different. Our expressions include:

- have a heart
- you're heartless
- he has a cold heart
- my heart aches
- I love you with all my heart

The Bible often mentions the word *heart* in both Old and New Testaments.

Part III of this book will show you how to improve emotional health using modern energy balancing techniques to reduce or eliminate emotional baggage and other bad energy. In effect, they heal the *heart*.

All types of energy affect bodily health. There is no way to remain healthy if the energies of our body, mind and spirit are unbalanced. Even when an individual's diet is healthy and alkalizing, mental and emotional stresses quickly make us acidic, negating our wise food choices.

Let's next see how ancient man viewed energy and healing.

**Ancient Energy Medicine**

Throughout history, man was deemed healthy when his energies—of body, mind *and* spirit—were balanced.

Problems originating with our body's energy eventually become physical problems. When energy is chaotic, the body will later gravitate toward physical pain, discomfort or illness.

If you are dehydrated, you drink water which contains energy. When you're hungry, you eat energizing food. Water and food are substances which contain energy. The energy healing methods mentioned in this book, however, deal primarily with what I call *pure* energy— such as heat, light, sound and magnetism.

One Chinese word for energy is *chi* which is included in the name of my Chi Choices website. This *chi* is the

*The Body and Energy*

energy that means we're alive. The medical people in ancient cultures viewed *chi* in various ways and we'll now briefly look at:

1. Traditional Chinese Medicine; and

2. Ayurvedic Medicine, also called Ayurveda, the medicine of ancient India.

Let's first look at *chi* in Traditional Chinese Medicine (TCM).

## TCM and Acupuncture Meridian Energy

Your entire body contains special energy points on energetic pathways. Energy flows up and down the body in acupuncture channels.

The ancient Chinese discovered 12 major acupuncture energy *rivers* in the body, called *meridians*, on which lie points of special energy. These points have been detected and verified using modern scientific instruments.

The Chinese saw two opposites everywhere, *yin* and *yang,* which need to be balanced using acupuncture needles, heat, herbs and other means. Half of the acupuncture meridians are *yin* meridians and the other half are *yang*. Half flow up the body and the rest flow down.

Each meridian contains what the ancient Chinese considered an *organ* of the body. We all have stomach, liver, heart, spleen, lung and other meridians. Various meridians go through the teeth, eyes, ears and tongue as well as through much of the body.

The manager of a health food store I knew had both a tooth and stomach problem. When I was in his store, I had a book with me that showed that his aching tooth was on the stomach meridian. He later told my wife he almost died due to a stomach infection. That stomach problem probably affected the tooth on the same meridian or perhaps a bad tooth resulted in stomach issues.

There are also two major *extraordinary vessels*. One of these is called the *governing vessel* or *governing meridian* and it is regularly used in one of the energy healing methods described in this book. The other is the *conception vessel*.

According to Traditional Chinese Medicine, when a person is sick, or about to become ill, the energy in meridians and vessels is problematic and out of balance. It can be too high, too low or confused. As we've seen, an acupuncture meridian can even flow backwards.

In addition to energetic points and meridians, let's now look at some large areas of energy within the body.

**Ayurveda and Chakra Energy**

Instead of *chi,* the people of India used the name *prana*. It has the same meaning—life giving or vital energy.

*The Body and Energy*

They saw energy in the body as tornado-like wheels of energy, which they called chakras, from the Sanskrit word *chakra,* meaning *wheel.* This energy resides in large energy centers within the body and which extend through and around the body horizontally.

There are 7 chakras between the tailbone and the top of the head. The lower 3 chakras are more related to the *body* and the material world. The top 4 chakras are associated with the *spiritual* world of mental, emotional and spiritual energy. There is also an eighth *chakra*—out there—away from the body.

Chakra energy can be measured today using ancient techniques as well as with modern electronic equipment. Chakras are a key part of Ayurvedic Medicine, the healing art of ancient India, which is still practiced today.

One important aim of Ayurvedic Medicine is to restore normal energy within the *chakras* of the body to achieve optimal health.

The energy healing techniques in Part III of this book either directly or indirectly tend to improve acupuncture and chakra energy, increasing the overall energy of the body, leading us to better health.

In the next chapter we'll delve into two windows into the subconscious mind—*muscle testing* and *intuition*—which will be used in the healing methods in Part III.

# Chapter Four

## SENSING ENERGY

Individuals are capable of detecting energy. Our body can communicate with us in various ways and some of them are used in the energy healing methods in Part III.

**Detecting Energy**

Alternative medical practitioners routinely examine parts of the body such as the eyes, tongue and fingernails to determine energetic harmony within us.

*Pure* energy, which I'll often just call energy, impacts the body and we can sometimes feel its vibrations. Take music. Its energy can affect us, positively or negatively.

Some people see the energy in the human aura, including chakra and acupuncture meridian energy, in living color. All of us can feel energy or vibrations when we're in a group of people or upon entering a room. Those *vibes* can be uplifting or depressing.

My grandfather knew how to sense and locate water. During the Great Depression, he found underground water by using a sapling.

Most scientists today do not know exactly how, or if, *water witching* works. Common sense tells me that nobody trains and pays a person during a depression to find water if it cannot be done. I asked my grandfather if he'd ever missed. He said one time they dug down and found only a buried water pipe.

In addition to sensing energy outside the body, such as in finding water, there are ways to measure energy within the body. One of these is called *muscle testing*.

**Muscle Testing and Stress**

What if you could ask your body what it needs or perhaps doesn't want—and get an answer? You probably can.

Your thoughts and words affect the strength of your muscles. Normally, your muscle strength will be:

- *stronger* when you say or think something *true* or *positive;* and

- *weaker* when you say or think something *false* or *negative.*

Let's assume your name is Nancy.

If you state, "My name is Nancy," which is true or say, "Unconditional love," which is positive, then your muscles will have a certain strength.

Conversely, if you state, "My name is William," or say, "Hatred," then *every* muscle in your body will become somewhat weaker because those statements are either not true or are negative. That causes stress, weakening muscles. This is the principle behind the *lie detector* test.

Muscle testing is a fascinating way to tap into your subconscious mind and inner wisdom and is often used by naturopathic doctors for nutritional testing. They use it to determine if your body needs a nutrient right now and, if so, which of several food supplements would be the best. It can also test for dosage.

Muscle testing is important because it usually allows us to tap into the subconscious mind. Sometimes we do *not* muscle test correctly. The most common reason is dehydration, usually solved by consuming water. Other reasons include neck problems and emotional upset.

Muscle testing is not perfect because sometimes the subconscious mind is reluctant to share information. It just likes to do its own thing to protect us from what it believes is greater harm. For example, people with cancer will often muscle test incorrectly—*even if* a biopsy has proven they do have cancer. Days or weeks later, they may muscle test accurately.

With one of the energy healing methods in Part III, muscle testing is used to determine if there's some emotion lodged in the body which the subconscious mind will allow to be released.

So how do we know if our muscles are strong or weak? Let's find out because several of the energy healing methods presented in this book *must* be done using muscle testing.

As for muscle testing, there are dozens of ways to perform it on ourselves or others. Some methods are described in *The Emotion Code*, a book by Dr. Bradley Nelson. Let's look at 2 of them: the *sway test* and the *arm test*.

**The Sway Test**

This is a method of muscle testing yourself which is usually done standing, looking straight ahead, with your feet apart. If energy is flowing properly, you will *sway* forward when stating a truthful response or something positive and *sway* backwards when stating something that is not true or is negative.

Plants grow toward sunlight and fish swim away from toxins. Similarly, humans lean *forward* toward truth and positives and *backwards* away from falsehoods and negatives. Many people can do the *sway test*, although some are better at it than others. For some, it may take several seconds to move strongly in the correct direction, but that's ok.

**The Arm Test**

One popular muscle testing method uses the arm. Let's say we have two people, Ann and Bill. Ann puts out one arm in front of her or to her side, palm down, and she attempts to keep her arm straight when Bill pushes on it.

Bill then pushes down on Ann's arm with steadily

increasing strength as Ann states, "My name is Ann." Bill pushes with several fingertips on the outside of Ann's wrist, just to the elbow side of the bump on the wrist. Since the statement is true, her arm remains strong.

If Ann then says, "My name is Bill," as Bill pushes down again, her arm will become slightly weaker. Some individuals become significantly weaker and their arm is easily pushed down.

By the way, this is not about strength. Let's reverse the roles. Even if Bill is a 300 pound football player and tries to keep his hand straight with moderate strength, Ann can easily push his arm down if he states something not true.

Now let's look at a different way of detecting energy.

## Intuition

Occasionally, we just know something without using our normal five senses. We use what is known as our *sixth sense,* often manifested as a hunch or a feeling in our gut. This is called *intuition*.

Intuition is useful. It can keep us from danger and assist us in making better decisions. We may have a feeling that we should go home a different way or skip the bank, then learn later that, had we driven our normal route or gone to the bank, we might have been in an auto accident or present during a bank robbery.

Intuition is sometimes called Extra Sensory Perception (ESP). We sense something *without* using our normal senses. Thoughts or images sometimes just pop into our head. We may see them or hear them, but not with our eyes or ears.

Once, when my family was struggling financially, the words "There's money in the mailbox" jumped into my mind while driving home from work. Sure enough, I found a totally unexpected check for over a hundred dollars in my mailbox.

Malcolm Gladwell wrote a fascinating book about intuition called *Blink*. His subtitle, *The Power of Thinking Without Thinking,* says it all. Intuition is not based on logical thinking. It just happens.

In the 1950s, José Silva discovered much about intuition. His book titled *The Silva Mind Control Method* relates how his young daughter, in a relaxed alpha brain wave state, became intuitive. He was helping her study as he'd done many times before, but one day was different.

His routine was to think of a question, ask it, then wait for his daughter to give him an answer. This particular day, to his amazement, she suddenly began to answer each question after he framed it his mind but *before* he spoke it. Using intuition, she was reading his mind.

Mr. Silva wrote to the famous Duke University ESP expert, Dr. J. B. Rhine, who had shown ESP was real—but only for some psychic people. Dr. Rhine downplayed the whole incident, implying that the girl had been psychic all along. Undaunted, Mr. Silva spent 10 years doing the same thing with 39 children

*Sensing Energy*

in his town of Laredo, Texas—with even better results.

Another daughter, Laura, stated that her father was eventually vindicated when a prestigious magazine reported that Dr. Rhine had stated that *everyone* is capable of intuition. Over the years, Mr. Silva taught about half a million people to become intuitive using his own methods.

There are various ways to enhance our intuitive abilities and practitioners of a few energy healing methods in this book use intuition. Whole books have been written on intuition and you may wish to explore them. However, most people find developing intuition is far more challenging than learning muscle testing.

**Reading People and Animals at a Distance**

Muscle testing and intuition are not limited by distance. Most of us have had an experience with intuition involving a distant person or event.

*Long distance* muscle testing, however, is a new concept for many, but it's easy to do. If you can muscle test yourself *in any manner,* such as using the *sway test,* then you are capable of muscle testing another person. Let's say your name is Mary and your friend Bob gives you permission to muscle test him.

When Mary muscle tests herself using any of the numerous self-testing methods, she says, "My name is Mary." If she tests strong, she knows she is muscle testing herself correctly.

She then thinks about muscle testing Bob and says,

"My name is Bob." It may take a few tries, but she will eventually test strong for Bob and weak for her own name.

In effect, *Mary is now Bob* and can use muscle testing on herself to tap into his Bob's subconscious wisdom. This long distance muscle testing can be done a foot away from Bob or thousands of miles away.

Energy healing methods using long distance muscle testing can be done on anyone, no matter where they are. They even work on animals. You need, of course, the permission of the individual or the owner of the animal.

Several healing methods described in Part III use long distance muscle testing methods or intuition.

We also showed that intuition is possible for everyone, but it is often very challenging to learn.

You do *not* need to be able to muscle test yourself or others to benefit from the energy healing techniques in Part III of this book. However, it is useful to be aware of their use and power.

We'll next examine healing with energy.

# Chapter Five

## ENERGY HEALING

Healing with energy is *not* new. *All* healing is really energy healing because everything is energy. As we've seen, the ancient Chinese and people of India believed that healing occurred when energy became better balanced.

We looked at some methods of detecting energy in the last chapter. Now let's investigate how we might use good energy to correct problematic energy within the body.

**Healing with Energy**

Man has used prayer, heat, acupuncture, sound, the mind, positive thinking, sunlight and numerous other energy healing methods to improve the health of the body over thousands of years. Let's look at heat and sound as examples of energetic healing.

**Heat.** American Indians use *sweat lodges* because heat kills pathogens and causes the body to eliminate toxins via perspiration. They wisely make use of the largest elimination organ of the body—the skin.

My Italian grandfather came to America in his early

teens because he had malaria and it was believed that a different climate might help him. When his malaria flared up on rare occasions, he took a hot bath, drank a little hard liquor, then went to bed. The extra heat from the bath and alcohol relieved his malaria symptoms overnight.

Today, when a patient has only a somewhat elevated temperature, some doctors try to knock it down. Other doctors, fortunately, believe the body knows best how to heal.

**Sound.** Sound has power and can heal or hurt. An opera singer can shatter a glass with her voice. Soldiers break step as they cross bridges because regular vibrations can intensify and collapse the bridge.

Loud music, lawnmowers and noisy machinery can damage our ears and increase our stress level. Rock band members either wear earplugs or suffer hearing loss. Pleasant music decreases stress. In the Bible, David was able to alleviate what is believed to be King Saul's depression by playing healing music on a lyre.

Sound affects our brain, chakras and the entire body. Andrew Weil, MD, and Kimba Arem give some good examples of that on their CD titled *Self-Healing with Sound and Music*.

Sharry Edwards, a sound healing expert, used sound to diagnose *and* reverse her own Parkinson's Disease. Another time, her son shattered his kneecap into 36 pieces in a motorcycle accident and was not expected to walk again. She used sound to heal him. In 10 weeks he was walking again with a completely regrown kneecap, as proven by an x-ray.

I heard those testimonies directly from Sharry Edwards. Her son's story is also detailed in *Vibrational Medicine,* a book of energy therapies by Richard Gerber, MD.

## Moving Energy

Albert Szent-Györgki, MD, PhD, won the Nobel Prize in 1937 for his discovery of Vitamin C. This brilliant scientist once said:

> In every culture and in every medical tradition before ours, healing was accomplished by moving energy.

What does he mean by *moving energy*? Well, the Chinese recently—make that some 5,000 years ago—developed a number of exercises that improve and move *chi* energy within the body. These exercises are called qigong. *Tai chi* uses some of the many qigong exercises. Every person who does *tai chi* knows about moving energy.

If energy healing is so great, do hospitals employ energy in actual healing? Some do, to a limited extent, such as using ultrasound to break up kidney stones. Even though hospitals rarely use only what the Chinese call *chi,* at least one does.

## A Hospital that Moves Energy

In China, the world's first medicineless hospital was

founded in 1988 by Pang Ming, MD, who is also a Qigong Grandmaster. In 1992, the hospital relocated to a city about 5 hours by train from Beijing. It is non-profit and the Chinese government regards it as a legitimate clinic.

In 2003, Luke Chan wrote about this hospital in a book titled *101 Miracles of Natural Healing*. It is the story of 101 people who, while patients at the hospital, recovered from arthritis, cancer, high blood pressure, diabetes, systemic lupus and from many diseases considered *incurable*.

Mr. Chan found so many people there healed of cancer that he stopped interviewing those whose cancer had been reversed. Many former patients volunteer at the hospital to give back to others.

Patients in this hospital take no medicine and have no unusual diets. They just perform special *qigong* energy moving exercises throughout the day and love is stressed. Patients can also receive *chi* from others.

Is moving *chi* energy beneficial? Absolutely! Mr. Chan mentions that this hospital had treated over 135,000 patients afflicted with some 180 different diseases. Its overall improvement rate was 95%. Only 5% of patients remained the same or got worse.

Furthermore, *chi* from other people can affect cancer tumors. Mr. Chan spent a month at the hospital in 1995. While there, he videotaped an ultrasonic display showing a large cancerous bladder tumor being shrunk with *chi* emitted by several hospital doctors. The cancerous tumor *disappeared* in less than a minute.

## Frequency and Healing

In Part I we mentioned that cellular health means our cells contain lots of *oxygen* and are slightly *alkaline*. Now let's add a third way of determining health—*frequency*.

Energy consists of frequencies. This is true of sound, light and solid substances because they move or are composed of smaller vibrating particles. If we measure the overall frequency of the body, a high frequency correlates with wellness while a lower one indicates sickness and ill health.

Harmful things, like bacteria, viruses and negative emotions all have low frequencies. Positive emotions have high frequencies. Our health, or lack thereof, is determined by all of our individual frequencies.

We learned earlier that Sharry Edwards healed her son's kneecap with sound. What did she do? She simply had him listen to the bone-building frequencies of calcium and magnesium from a special computer. Those *sounds* repaired his knee.

How was that possible? Well, every *solid* substance, including human bone, is made of atoms, which are really just frequencies. Listening to them puts those frequencies into the body. Even if we cannot hear all the frequencies, they still affect us.

Much more information about music, sound, color and frequency healing is contained in the book *Secret*

*Sounds* by Jill Mattson. The first part of the book is the story of Sharry Edwards.

Let's look at the effect of words.

Substances like water, for example, can be affected by various frequencies, even by words and thoughts.

Dr. Masaru Emoto is a Japanese man who exposes water to various energies, then freezes the water, forming ice crystals. Dirty water or water exposed to negative words or thoughts, such as *hatred*, produce ugly and distorted water crystals.

Water exposed to positive words, such as *unconditional love* create beautiful crystals. Dr. Emoto determined that the high frequency words of *love* and *gratitude*—combined—produced the most perfectly formed ice crystals. Gratitude is related to positive thinking where we are grateful to see a water glass as half full, not half empty.

In his book *Power vs. Force,* David Hawkins, MD, has a scale of energies, derived via muscle testing. His lowest energy level is *shame*, which is highly damaging. Dr. Hawkins believes that people at this level are prone to psychosis, paranoia and suicide, as well as to committing bizarre crimes.

At the other end of his spectrum is *enlightenment*. Dr. Hawkins mentions that only a few people attain this high frequency state—people like Jesus Christ and Buddha and a handful of others. The rest of us lie somewhere between *shame* and *enlightenment*.

In his book *Think and Grow Rich,* Napoleon Hill mentions that prayers said with positive thoughts and emotions work best. If we pray with fear and doubt then our prayers may not be as effective, since we are sending out prayers mixed with low frequencies. When we mix positive high frequency emotions with prayer, in faith, good things often result.

Now let's examine how thoughts can be focused and directed at others.

## Intention and the Conscious Mind

We've already discussed the power of habits and beliefs in our subconscious mind. However, the conscious mind is also important in energy healing. When we focus our thoughts, that is known as *intention.*

Intention is an incredibly powerful force—for better or worse. The human mind is designed as a goal seeking computer. Most people intend to do good, with love, to help their family and others. Others, with evil intent, commit crimes of theft, extortion, murder and even genocide.

The mental energy of intention is potent. We can just think about getting sick and often that is exactly what happens. We can also envision ourselves finding some way to heal a problematic condition and that often occurs.

Our subconscious mind may cause us to seek out novel ways to improve our health. That thinking may be what drew you to this book.

**Intention, Epigenetics and DNA**

Intention affects us far more than our DNA. Take identical twins with the same education and talents. One succeeds admirably and one fails miserably at the same job. Why? Well, maybe one of them had a stronger intention to succeed than the other. But, there can be other reasons.

Furthermore, why do the life spans of identical twins often differ by 15 years, despite having the *same* genes and DNA? The answer is that *environment* is more important than genes. As they say, "DNA is not destiny."

All stimuli, sensed by the cell membrane, ultimately influence our DNA. Anything with a frequency impacts our DNA. This includes our thoughts, beliefs, stress, trauma, images and emotions. Remember, we just discussed the importance of frequency to health.

The problem is that most people, including doctors, don't understand or haven't heard of *epigenetics*—the study of how genes get turned on and off by biological forces *outside* our DNA. It is a new and largely unknown science.

If more people understood epigenetics, they would be more receptive to diet, exercise and other healthy living practices that effect our DNA. They would focus more on eliminating low frequency stressors, including stress and trauma, behind cancer and most diseases. They would also think positively and realize that negative emotions and thinking do far more damage than harmful genes that may never be *expressed*.

Genes in our DNA are like light switches. They can be off or on. We want to have good genes *expressed*, that is, turned on, and bad genes *silenced*, that is, turned off. This is accomplished in several ways, including winding or unwinding our DNA and covering or uncovering sections of DNA with a protein sheath. A covered gene cannot be expressed. It's like a light that's off with the light switch hidden so nobody can find it to turn it on.

Dr. Peter D'Adamo, famous for his *blood type diet* books, wrote a later book titled The *GenoType Diet*. It has these words on the cover: *your personalized plan for turning off the bad genes and turning on the good ones*. It's all about epigenetics and health.

Some people believe that possessing a certain breast cancer gene will automatically result in breast cancer. This faulty belief and lack of positive intention could actually make it come true. Some women with such a gene have even undergone mastectomies—without having cancer. How sad and tragic it is that they and their doctors were ignorant of epigenetics and the power of intention.

In energy healing, intention is used to seek a beneficial outcome for yourself or for another, based on love and concern. That kind of mental focus can produce wonderful healing outcomes. Many of the healing techniques in Part III use that kind of intention.

## Walking with Intention

We've already seen that rote tasks involve the subconscious mind. However, it is possible, using intention, to perform them consciously, but it takes a great deal of mental work and focus. John Pepper, a man in South Africa, taught himself to do exactly that. Mr. Pepper has been able to walk close to 4 miles an hour, or more, over many years. That's fast for a healthy person and incredible for Mr. Pepper, a man with Parkinson's Disease.

People with Parkinson's Disease are low in dopamine, a neurotransmitter, in part of their brain. Lack of dopamine causes them to struggle with movement and often experience tremors. But, Mr. Pepper taught himself and others to walk, eat and drink *consciously* —without tremors—by using intent and thinking about each minute movement.

Intrigued by Mr. Pepper, Norman Doidge, MD, a Canadian psychiatrist and brain neuroplasticity expert, traveled to South Africa to meet with Mr. Pepper and his neurologist. Mr. Pepper's story is described in *The Brain's Way of Healing*, a book written later by Dr. Doidge.

Conscious thinking uses a different part of the brain which contains ample dopamine. Mr. Pepper's story demonstrates that intention is so powerful that it can bypass the subconscious mind.

## Energy Healing Principles

Energy healing improves energy within the body, which leads to better health. Traditional Chinese Medicine seeks to improve and balance *yin* and *yang* energy in the body. Ayurvedic Medicine seeks to improve energy in the chakras of the body.

The healing methods in Part III of this book primarily use *pure* energy to help the body heal.

Energy balancing and healing involves:

1. identifying low frequency energy problems, often using *muscle testing* and *intuition*; and

2. balancing energy in the body, often using *intention*, magnets, light and *chi* energy to bring the body into greater harmony.

When we raise the overall frequency of our body, we become healthier. This is accomplished whenever we eliminate low frequency problems such as negative thoughts and emotions. The rest of this book will introduce you to many methods of doing that.

## Distant Healing

We all know that intuition commonly involves a distant person or event. We also saw in the last chapter that long distance muscle testing is possible. Intention also works from afar. So, energy healing can sense or even change energy in another person who can be next to us or on the other side of the earth.

This is all possible because everything is *energetically*

connected and there are many scientific ways to prove that.

For example, two electrons or two samples of DNA that have been in contact and then separated maintain their connection—at any distance. If a change is made to one of them, the other changes *instantly*—even if one of them had been sent into space. They are not talking to each other. Rather, they are still *connected,* albeit in some mysterious manner within the realm of quantum physics.

Therefore, many forms of energy healing can be performed at a distance because muscle testing, intuition and intention can all function regardless of distance. These long distance *tools* are necessary for many of the energy healing methods presented next in Part III of this book.

In the next part of this book, you'll be introduced to 6 powerful healing methods using energy which most doctors have never heard of. Some of them can work almost immediately while others take longer.

# Part III

# ENERGY HEALING SOLUTIONS

In Part I, we met the terrible twins—*stress* and *trauma*. They gang up on us to steal our oxygen, injure our immune system, upset us emotionally, terrorize our internal neighborhood, cause us grief and deliver pain and disease.

In Part II, we linked health with the energies of our body, mind, thoughts, spirit and emotions. We discussed the *tools* of muscle testing, intuition and intention which are often used in energy healing and which will be used in some of the methods we'll now discuss.

This portion of the book—Part III—will show you 6 ways to balance your body's energies, increase cellular oxygen and boost your immune system. These modern healing modalities also deal with emotional stress and trauma—often permanently—which can reduce pain and correct illness. These healing methods are:

## 6 LIFE CHANGING ENERGY HEALING METHODS

1. The Emotional Freedom Techniques (EFT)
2. The Emotion Code
3. The Healing Code
4. Biophoton Therapy
5. Craniosacral Therapy
6. The Original Chi Machine

At the end of this book, there is a *Resources Appendix* which will assist you with many of these healing techniques.

# Chapter Six

## PERFORM EMOTIONAL ACUPUNCTURE WITHOUT NEEDLES

Acupuncture points can be stimulated with needles, heat and electricity, as well as by rubbing them and tapping on them.

Let's say you're in intense physical or emotional pain, so you say a few words, tap on some acupuncture points with your fingers and become pain free in a few minutes. That's not only possible, but I've done it numerous times—for myself and others.

**The Emotional Freedom Techniques (EFT)**

For many years, I've used a tapping technique called the Emotional Freedom Techniques (EFT), which is used by millions. It is sometimes called *Acupuncture Without Needles* because acupuncture points are tapped but no needles are used

EFT is one of many techniques for reducing stress, pain and discomfort by tapping on some of the body's acupuncture points. Saying some words and tapping acupuncture points has been shown to help normalize or balance energy within the body, especially related to the problem being verbalized.

In my state, I was probably the first one to receive both basic and advanced EFT certificates, in 2007, as they had to add Mississippi to put me on their list. My specialty is using EFT to quickly reduce or eliminate physical pain.

EFT is easy to do and learn, at least for routine stress and pain. I once did EFT with a lady in a physical therapy office and her headache was gone in about a minute. She then went down the hall, met someone else with a headache, did EFT on her, and the other person's headache also disappeared.

Let's look at how EFT began.

**Origins of EFT**

In the 1980s, an American psychologist, Roger Callahan, PhD, a specialist in anxiety disorders, was working with a lady who was deathly afraid of water. Even touching water caused her to panic.

After more than a year, he'd made little progress with her. One day she announced, for the first time, that her fear was in her stomach. Dr. Callahan, in doing whatever he did that day, had her tap under her eye on an acupuncture point he knew to be on the stomach acupuncture meridian.

To his utter amazement, the lady stated that her fear of water had disappeared and, to prove it, she ran outside to a swimming pool, splashed water on her face and began laughing. Dr. Callahan determined that her fear of water was permanently gone.

After that experience, Dr. Callahan developed a method called Thought Field Therapy (TFT). TFT involves tapping acupuncture points while thinking, for example, of a fear. He developed a complicated TFT protocol which involved tapping acupuncture points in specific sequences. TFT is still used today as a healing art.

Dr. Callahan started teaching TFT to others, one of whom was a Stanford educated engineer in California named Gary Craig. In 1993, Mr. Craig developed the Emotional Freedom Techniques (EFT), a simpler cousin of TFT. Unlike TFT, EFT needs no special tapping algorithms.

Mr. Craig, founder of EFT, compares physical and emotional problems and stresses in the body to static on the radio. EFT seeks to remove this energetic racket from the body.

Traditional Chinese Medicine and Indian Ayurvedic Medicine view sickness and disease as energetic imbalances and blockages within the body. *Emotional acupuncture*—EFT—often corrects those conditions.

What does EFT work on? Mr. Craig says to try it on *everything*. He and others have used EFT to reverse PTSD and hundreds of other conditions related to stress and trauma.

EFT has been used to eliminate traumatic *war memories* for veterans in days or weeks that conventional one-on-one psychological therapy could not reverse over decades. Later in this chapter we'll see how EFT reversed trauma and multiple sclerosis in one individual.

**Proof of EFT Effectiveness**

EFT has been shown to be highly effective over many years for a variety of reasons. Here are some of them.

**Reason 1: Clients report that EFT works.** Skeptics say it's only due to the placebo effect because clients *think* it will help them. That's easily proven incorrect because EFT works on infants and animals who are *not* thinking of getting better or having less pain.

**Reason 2: EFT Changes Human Blood.** One EFT practitioner showed her doctor that she was able, in a few minutes, to use EFT to change her clumped up sluggish blood. This was shown to be the case because her doctor took *before* and *after* blood samples and examined them under a dark field microscope.

The red blood cells *before* EFT were clumped up. But her blood, *after* only a few minutes of EFT, done *specifically* for the purpose of correcting the clumped blood, was able to flow freely, carrying much more oxygen. Photos of this phenomenon are shown by Dawson Church, PhD, in his book titled *The Genie in your Genes*.

**Reason 3: Doctors Use EFT.** Some doctors, like Dr. Joseph Mercola and Dr. Eric Robins, use EFT and teach it to their patients. Doctors say there are no EFT side effects, which is not true for *any* pharmaceutical drug.

Dr. Mercola is an osteopathic physician whose enormous website contains information and videos on just about every wellness topic, including EFT. At different times, I met two individuals who had traveled from Mississippi to Illinois to see him. He healed them both when their local doctor could not, so I know he has excellent patient references.

Dr. Robins is a urologist who also uses EFT with his patients. He is also featured in an excellent EFT video on the EFT website.

I did EFT on several occasions with a friend who was a chiropractic doctor. The first time we did EFT, his pain went away quickly so he asked for EFT again the next time we met because he knew it worked.

Some physical therapists use EFT with patients experiencing pain or having mobility issues. I took an EFT class with a physical therapist who was already using it when therapy was not working and the patient's insurance was running out. He had helped many patients for whom physical therapy *alone* was just not the answer.

**EFT Basics**

To do EFT, you think of a specific *problem* while tapping acupuncture points. This procedure often results in a reduction of emotional or physical pain, fears, phobias and jet lag. EFT can often improve your golf score, eyesight or hundreds of other conditions of pain and illness.

EFT works when there is no *psychological reversal*—a condition in which we are our own worst enemies and find our conscious and subconscious minds fighting each other. EFT uses the *setup* technique which, at least temporarily, can undo psychological reversal before performing the EFT tapping sequence.

There are only two basic emotions: *love* and *fear*. EFT, in its purest form, frees us from our negative emotions and thought patterns by replacing low frequency *fear* with high frequency *love*. It employs the physiological technique, known as a *reframe*, in which a negative *fear* such as anxiety, dread or anger is replaced with positive *love*.

Here are some basic steps for doing EFT for a pain issue:

**Step 1: Identify your pain problem.** Let's assume it's a pain in your right elbow.

**Step 2: Determine your initial pain level for that specific pain.** The pain level is from 0–10, with 0 being no distress or pain and 10 being maximum pain.

**Step 3: Determine your *setup* phrase.** Be specific, so if your right elbow hurts, for your setup, you might want to say, "Even though I have right elbow pain, I deeply and completely *love* and accept myself."

Or you might prefer to say, "Even though my right

elbow hurts, I deeply and completely accept myself."

**Step 4: Select a *reminder* phrase.** Your reminder phrase is something that reminds you of your problem. As a reminder of your problem, you might say, "Right elbow pain."

**Step 5: State the setup statement out loud (or to yourself) while tapping on the heel of your hand.** The place you hit is the part of the hand used for a karate chop. Tap the heel of one hand on the *karate chop* point with several fingers of the other hand or with the heel of the other hand. Continue tapping until you have said the setup statement 3 times.

**Step 6: Tap several acupuncture points, one at a time, while saying out loud (or to yourself) the reminder phrase once on each point.** For the above issue of right elbow pain, while tapping each point, you say, "Right elbow pain."

There are 8 tapping points described below. Each location is tapped about half a dozen times while repeating the reminder phrase. The number of times is not critical. The important thing is repeating the reminder phrase once for each point to keep the problem *on your mind* while you're tapping that point.

EFT works when the problem is on your mind *and* you are tapping an acupuncture point.

**Step 7: Determine your final distress or pain level for your specific pain.** If your distress level is not zero then you can repeat steps one through seven. If your pain level has dropped, add the word *remaining* to your reminder phrase so, while tapping each point, you will say, "Remaining right elbow pain."

Pain sometimes moves so if you find that the pain in your right elbow is now somewhere else, change your setup statement. If the pain is now in your right wrist, simply do the second round of tapping and say, "Right wrist pain" as your modified reminder phrase.

If you have done about 5 rounds of EFT and still have pain, it is best to stop. I'll give some additional tips in this chapter about what to do when EFT does not seem to be working very well.

**EFT Tapping Points**

Let's now look at points often tapped during EFT. For each point, you'll see the acupuncture meridian or extraordinary vessel on which that point is located. Many points are found on both sides of the body so, for them, either one can be used.

The setup point and the first 8 points are used by Mr. Craig in a fairly recent YouTube video titled *The Basic EFT Recipe*. Unless mentioned, most points are commonly tapped with the index and middle fingers as it is easier to hit the correct spot with at least 2 fingers.

Here are the EFT tapping points:

**The setup point (small intestine meridian).**

This is in the middle of the heel of the hand, the karate chop point.

The next 8 points are used following the setup procedure.

**Point 1: Top of the head.** This is on the top, back fairly flat portion of the head, on a line between the nose and the back of the neck. This is usually tapped with 4 fingers or with the palm of the hand. All meridians go through this point.

**Point 2: End of the eyebrow (bladder meridian).** This is on the end of the eyebrow, near the nose.

**Point 3: Side of the eye (gallbladder meridian).** This is on the side of the eye, on the bone of the eye socket, near the ear.

**Point 4: Under the eye (stomach meridian).** This is under the eye on the bone of the eye socket.

**Point 5: Under the nose (governing vessel).** This is between the nose and upper lip.

**Point 6: Chin area (conception vessel).** This point is under the lower lip in the indentation at the top of the chin.

**Point 7: Collarbone bump (kidney meridian).** This is the bump where the collarbone ends as it drops down near the front base of the neck.

**Point 8: Under the arm (spleen meridian).** This is about 4 inches below the armpit. If you put one arm across your chest and parallel to the ground, then tap with 4 fingers, you'll hit the right spot. You can also slap your hand under your armpit.

Acupuncture meridians *communicate* with each other so it is not mandatory to use points on each meridian. The following points are on other meridians or are special points that some people, including myself, regularly use:

**Point 9. Base of the breast (liver meridian).** This is under the breast, directly below the nipple, in the same location for men and women.

**Point 10: Inside of the wrist.** This can be tapped with several fingers or with the other wrist. Multiple meridians go through this special wrist area.

**Points 11–15: Fingers.** They may be tapped together, all at once, with corresponding fingertips touching each other.

They may also be tapped one at a time. When tapped individually by a right handed person, the index finger and middle finger of the right hand connect with the flesh just to the right of each fingernail on the left hand when the left hand is pointing upwards. A left handed person does the opposite.

Here is some information about individual fingers.

**Point 11: Thumb (lung meridian).**

**Point 12: Index finger (large intestine meridian).**

**Point 13: Middle finger (pericardium meridian).**

**Point 14: Ring finger (triple warmer meridian).**

**Point 15: Baby finger (heart meridian).** We tap on this point on the side of the nail nearest to the thumb. The baby finger also contains the small intestine meridian which is on the opposite side of the baby finger and which goes though the karate chop point on the heel of the hand.

**Point 16: Ankle area.** This point is located in the soft spot on the inside of the foot between the ankle bone and the back of the foot. This can be tapped with several fingers. Multiple meridians go through this special ankle area.

**When EFT is Not Working**

EFT issues may have different aspects. If so, working on additional aspects of the problem is the next step. Mr. Craig compares aspects to the legs of a table. If a table has many legs, you don't have to saw off all the legs before the table falls. Likewise, a problem with multiple aspects will often be resolved after several aspects have been handled with EFT.

Apart from aspects, Mr. Craig tells us that there are special circumstances when EFT will *not* work. This is true for clients with severe polarity or psychological reversals, food allergies or those affected by toxins.

I did EFT on a friend with no results and later found

out that he was a Hurricane Katrina victim who, after Katrina, was living upstairs in a flooded house with mold downstairs. He was affected by toxic mold.

When I first started doing EFT, my disappointments exceeded my successes, leading me to spend hours on the EFT website. I started taking notes from most of my sessions to learn from them. The 4 things that helped the most were:

1. saying a silent prayer, before or during the session, such as, "Lord, help me assist this person;"

2. believing my EFT skills could help *anyone* in pain;

3. using *both* sides of the body and individual fingers after any unsuccessful round of tapping; and

4. tapping for the emotional stress *behind* the physical pain when tapping for the physical pain no longer seems to work.

Sometimes I tap on myself and let the client mimic me or, with their permission, I tap on them. We usually use all or most of the 16 points described above.

If the client wants me to tap on their body, the client still taps corresponding fingers together and, if used, the liver point under the breast. I tap the rest of the points, including individual fingers if we are using them. Occasionally we omit the liver point under the breast and don't use the ankle point if the client is wearing boots.

Here are my 3 current methods for performing EFT for *pain*, my specialty:

## Method 1: Normal tapping.

I normally use all or most of the 16 points described above for the first round of tapping—using one side of the body. I let the client tap corresponding fingers together because it's much faster than using individual fingers.

If there is a marked change in pain level I use the same points on subsequent rounds. It typically takes about 2–4 rounds to get to 0.

If there is no pain level change or if it is minimal, like a 10 only dropping to a 9, then I take extraordinary measures on subsequent rounds to try to relieve the pain quickly.

## Method 2: Extraordinary tapping.

I normally use *all* the points above on *both sides* of the body until the pain level is gone or no longer dropping.

The reason we do this is because sometimes there is a blockage on one side of the body that prevents energy from moving properly. By tapping on both sides, we can often bypass the energy roadblock. Remember, points on the vertical centerline of the body, such as the top of the head, do not have a second point to tap so we only tap the one point.

## Method 3: Looking behind the pain

When the pain level does not change or changes minimally over several rounds, I try to determine the emotional stress *behind* their pain. I often ask, "Is there some stress in your life now that might be contributing to your pain?"

People know their stresses—relationship issues, the unfair boss, driving to work in heavy traffic, financial issues, or any number of daily stresses and strains. Subsequent tapping for their most stressful emotional problem usually reduces the physical pain along with their emotional stress.

## Mental EFT

EFT, like many energy healing methods, can be done in your mind. You say the EFT words silently and imagine tapping each acupuncture point. Mental tapping works as well as physical tapping according to Mr. Craig, the founder of EFT, and I agree.

I used to tap on my body on airplanes for *jet lag* and little kids would look at me and wonder what this strange man was doing. Once, as a test, when my wife and I were on an airplane returning from a visit to our daughter in England, I tapped *only* mentally every few hours for jet lag. It worked just as well as physical tapping.

Mental tapping is also convenient for those with problems using their hands such as people in meetings as well as those with tremors or confined to bed.

## Long Distance EFT

We discussed healing at a distance in the last chapter. The name for this in the EFT world is *surrogate* EFT. The client obviously needs to give their permission, as they do for any other session. *Surrogate* EFT has also been used on animals.

To do *surrogate* or long distance EFT, you use intent, that is, you focus your thoughts strongly on your client. You could also use muscle testing to connect with them as I now do. You can then do EFT *on their behalf* by:

1. tapping *physically* on yourself; or

2. tapping *mentally* on either yourself or on them.

All of these will work because intention is the key. You can use intuition or muscle testing to gauge how you are doing or, when possible, you simply ask the client.

## EFT Results

EFT has helped reverse, or make better, these and other conditions:

- addictions, anxiety, athletic performance,
- bee stings, cravings, depression, discomfort,
- emotional pain and stress, fears, jet lag,

- multiple sclerosis (and other serious diseases),
- Obsessive Compulsive Disorder (OCD),
- numbness, phobias, physical aches and pain, PTSD,
- some terminal illnesses, surgery prevention,
- tremors, vision problems and weight loss.

Let's now look at how EFT eliminated a so-called *incurable* disease.

**EFT Reverses Multiple Sclerosis**

Hank Hadley fell down a hay chute at age 10, landing on his tailbone on concrete. This and other accidents led to many operations, excruciating pain, pain pills and addiction to numerous pain medications. He suffered much trauma and also developed multiple sclerosis.

The introductory video on the EFT website tells a little of Hank's story although the video calls him Harry. He had been on Social Security disability for years and had been five years in and out of a wheelchair prior to EFT.

EFT allowed Hank to start using crutches again. In a few months he did *jumping jacks* in the office of his EFT therapist. His EFT recovery took a very long time, with lots of setbacks, despite Hank tapping regularly.

Eventually, he ended up functioning well, off disability, working in his own outdoor business—and

—his multiple sclerosis is gone. His remaining addiction is EFT.

**Personal EFT Experiences**

I have used EFT on friends and family for over a decade with mostly positive results in several hundred sessions. I'll now discuss a few EFT successes and experiences I've had.

If my client wants to do the tapping, I first let the client find and practice tap each point ahead of the actual tapping. But, they practice tap only *after* they tell me their pain level because just tapping sometimes reduces their pain.

Sometimes the client *feels* some sensation within the body while tapping. For example, I've had several people report they felt something in their stomach when tapping the stomach meridian acupuncture point under the eye—the same point Dr. Roger Callahan used with the lady mentioned earlier who was suffering from fear of water. Another client felt something in her heart when tapping her pinkie which is on the heart meridian.

**EFT for Hurricane Katrina Trauma.** In 2005, Hurricane Katrina flooded and partially destroyed our home, as I've already stated.

After Katrina, we stayed about a week with friends in Texas. From there, my mother and one of our daughters flew to different states to stay with relatives. My wife I returned to Mississippi about a week later and rented a different house.

Everything was chaos and EFT was fairly new to me, so I didn't even think about trying it until returning to Mississippi. After that, I did EFT on myself a number of times and I've never had a negative feeling when discussing Hurricane Katrina.

On the other hand, one of my wife's relatives, after Katrina, told us about his family's experiences during Hurricane Camille over 35 years earlier. He became emotional while recalling how floodwaters inside their home had forced him and his family into their attic during the storm.

**EFT for Back Pain.** Back problems have bothered me for decades, starting in the 1960s, but they rarely occur now. Over many decades, I've had my back adjusted, using many different techniques, by chiropractors in several states, Japan and Canada.

A low back problem that would once plague me for about 5 days is now usually gone in a few minutes through the use of EFT. I've also gotten great results from getting Craniosacral Therapy and using the Chi Machine, both discussed later in this book.

I'm very sympathetic to those with back pain. So, when a lady in her early 70s approached me after a Wednesday night Mass and told me that her back hurt, I offered to try EFT with her.

Her initial pain level was 5. In the church parking lot, I did the tapping on her, using the reminder statement of *mid back pain,* which she repeated aloud. We did one round of tapping, which took about a minute, after which she was pain free.

We then did an optional procedure known as a *floor-to-ceiling eye roll* which takes about 7 seconds. I felt it might cement things even more. Often that procedure can quickly reduce a pain level of 1 or 2 to 0. I have also successfully used it for pain levels of 3. In the *Resources Appendix,* there is a short video showing how to perform the floor-to-ceiling eye roll.

This lady later told my mother that her back had been getting progressively worse over the months before our EFT session and that she had no idea as to what kind of doctor might be able to help her. She has now been free of back pain for many years—after less than 2 minutes of EFT.

**EFT for Excruciating Pain.** A friend living in another state called me on the telephone. He told me he had a lot of pain under his right breast, due to a fall near his swimming pool. He was recovering from left shoulder surgery so when he fell he twisted his upper body in order to avoid landing on his bad side.

He agreed to try EFT over the telephone. We had done EFT in person in the past, so he knew a little about EFT. I told him where to tap and what to say.

When asked for his initial pain level, he said, "Excruciating," which I took as a 10. Several rounds of EFT reduced it to 5, then to 0. We did a floor-to-ceiling eye roll as insurance. This man went from excruciating pain to no pain in about 6 minutes.

**Traumatic Memories Gone.** Over 5 years ago, I used EFT to erase some traumatic memories that my mom had experienced in high school—some 70 years earlier. They all disappeared in about 15–20 minutes. The emotion associated with them has never returned.

**EFT Quick Results.** I have seen many issues partially or totally resolved in one session of EFT. These include physical pain such as headaches, back and neck pain, as well as stress, phobias, fears, anxiety and emotional upset. However, each situation is different and some may take numerous sessions to handle.

**EFT Advantages**

People use EFT all over the world because it is simple to do and no equipment is needed. You can do EFT yourself and even mentally. You can also do EFT with a practitioner in person or over the telephone. EFT can also be done for you—even long distance—using surrogate EFT.

Most problems, when they have been *properly* addressed by an experienced EFT practitioner, will *not* come back, according to Mr. Craig. That is also my experience.

**EFT Limitations**

Tremendous skill is needed to handle serious psychological situations as well as difficult and complex situations involving serious diseases, depression, Post Traumatic Stress Disorder (PTSD) and addictions.

# # #

See the *Resources Appendix* for more information about EFT. It will also show you how to find an EFT practitioner who can work with you in person, on the telephone or with an internet program like Skype or FaceTime.

# Chapter Seven

## EXPEL AN EMOTION WITH A REFRIGERATOR MAGNET

Emotions stuck or trapped in the body are most difficult to release by traditional medical methods such as talk therapy. Fortunately, they can quickly and easily be removed, one at a time, using intention and a refrigerator magnet.

This unusual emotion zapping method is named *The Emotion Code*.

**The Emotion Code**

Emotions *do* affect the body. They cause physical symptoms such as blushing, a dry mouth, tightness in the stomach or a racing pulse.

The Emotion Code is an energy balancing technique developed by Dr. Bradley Nelson, a chiropractic doctor who is a world famous energy healer and medical intuitive. He loves to work with so-called *incurable* conditions. His method is designed to identify, then release harmful emotions which are lodged in the body.

In 2007, Dr. Nelson wrote a book titled *The Emotion Code*. It deals with emotional stress and trauma due to what he coined *Trapped Emotions,* a name I'll use in this chapter.

Dr. Nelson wrote the book so his readers could learn to release stuck emotions from themselves and others. He also states that no specific Trapped Emotion, once released, has *ever* returned.

**Trapped Emotions**

In Part I, we saw that destructive negative emotions become lodged *inside* the body's tissues if they are not handled correctly. The average person possesses several hundred of them. Children often have far fewer than adults. Now let's explore how emotions might get embedded in the body.

Let's say we get angry when a distracted driver cuts us off on the road. When that energy of anger is raging, other previously trapped anger emotions, both our own and inherited ones, become activated. They resonate with our current anger, making things much worse. Perhaps this is one cause of road rage.

Some of us may pray for the other driver or say, "I guess he's having a bad day" and that emotion of anger disappears, never remaining permanently in the body. Other people get all upset, dwell on the incident or even try to chase down the bad driver.

Some Trapped Emotions are inherited from our ancestors and others we generate ourselves.

**Inherited Trapped Emotions.** We *inherit* some Trapped Emotions like we inherit our eye or hair color. *Inherited* Trapped Emotions come to us, without our permission, from our parents. Most of them originated with them or with our grandparents, but some do come from earlier ancestors.

Trapped Emotions can be passed on to one, all or none of our children.

**Personal Trapped Emotions.** Most Trapped Emotions *really* are our own. They got trapped or stuck in us *after* we were born. We experience an emotion and, if it's not dealt with adequately, it takes up residence somewhere in the body, often in a location that has been weakened in the past.

Some emotions we pick up or *absorb* from another person near us, often from family or friends who are experiencing some intense emotion. We can also absorb them from the radio, television, a movie or video.

In a riot or demonstration, participants often experience the same emotions. They are probably absorbing the negative emotions from others in the group.

**Prenatal Trapped Emotions.** A baby in the womb is capable of generating an emotion once the organ which creates that emotion is formed in the fetus. It may also *absorb* an emotion from its mother, father or sibling.

Trapped Emotions can occur in a baby in the womb

throughout pregnancy, but this happens mostly during the third trimester.

I know one person who had a number of prenatal Trapped Emotions which muscle testing revealed had gotten trapped during the second trimester. He then volunteered the information that his father had left his mother in the middle of her pregnancy which would certainly affect his mother directly and him, indirectly, due to *absorbed* emotions.

This client did the muscle testing for this session himself, using the *sway test,* which he could easily do. However, the sway test takes a lot of time, so most practitioners, including myself, prefer to do the muscle testing ourselves *on behalf of* the client to save time. I prefer a 2-finger method, using only one hand, which is called the *hand solo* method.

**Groups of Trapped Emotions.** Sometimes, several Trapped Emotions—usually 2 or 3—are stored together. The subconscious mind usually wants to release *all* the Trapped Emotions in one of these groups at the same time.

When several Trapped Emotions are located together in the same area of the body, the word *nested* is used to refer to these emotions.

Some groups of Trapped Emotions, generated by one traumatic event, are stored in a single ball of energy. Such a grouping is called a P*sychic Trauma.* Psychic Traumas were discovered after the terrorist events of 9–11 when many people experienced several intense emotions simultaneously.

**Heart-Wall Emotions.** Around the heart is a huge electromagnetic field, which extends many feet out from the body and touches those around us. We know that it is possible to be in a room and feel *good vibes* or *bad vibes* coming from the hearts of others.

Sometimes we wall in that heart. Most people (about 93%), including some children, have what Dr. Nelson calls a Heart-Wall, which is *constructed* of various kinds of Trapped Emotions we've just described. These Trapped Emotions form a protective energetic barrier around the heart.

The Heart-Wall collapses when the Trapped Emotion building blocks are released, often improving one's peace, health and life. Most Trapped Emotions in the body are not part of the Heart-Wall. However, a portion of our pain and discomfort can be tied to a Heart-Wall.

Fortunately, a Heart-Wall can be cleared of Trapped Emotions using the Emotion Code procedures.

**Destructive Trapped Emotions**

Each Trapped Emotion is a *ball of energy* located in *one* particular part of the body, perhaps in the stomach, low back or elbow. The part of the body where it resides is often a weaker part of the body, perhaps one injured in the past or weakened by some stress.

If we've suffered an injury to our left knee, Trapped

Emotions may be stored there in preference to the right knee. Eventually we may have problems with our left knee while our right knee appears normal. If a doctor later tells us we need a left knee replacement, it should come as no surprise.

Trapped Emotions are *foreign* to the body and are a source of irritation and energy disruption to the tissues of the body. Dr. Nelson says they often range from the size of an orange to that of a cantaloupe. Unless released, they can eventually cause health issues and disease.

The body's healing system—the immune system—and our organs and glands often do not work normally when we are under the stress of Trapped Emotions. This stress leads to inflammation, fatigue, discomfort, pain, illness and disease as Dr. Hans Selye, the *Father of Stress,* discovered.

Many common phobias, such as fears of elevators, heights, being closed in, flying, public speaking and many others, can be seriously debilitating. Dr. Nelson believes that phobias are caused largely by Trapped Emotions and possibly only by them.

**Releasing Trapped Emotions**

It's possible to release Trapped Emotions from others, with their permission, or from yourself using The Emotion Code provided that you have learned to do muscle testing, which is explained in great detail in the book.

Assuming you can muscle test yourself, or have a

## Expel an Emotion with a Refrigerator Magnet

friend who can do it for you, how do you release a Trapped Emotion affecting some pain or health issue you have? How do you clear a Heart-Wall?

Well, for each of these procedures, you simply follow a flowchart and use a chart of 60 Trapped Emotions. These charts are found in *The Emotion Code* book written by Dr. Nelson. Dr. Nelson has 2 flowcharts in his book, one for clearing normal Trapped Emotions and another for releasing those in the Heart-Wall.

With some practice, using muscle testing, most people can find—and permanently release—a Trapped Emotion or a Heart-Wall emotion in a minute or two. Powerful magnets, or even weak refrigerator magnets, are often used to magnify our intention needed to release the Trapped Emotion.

However, magnets should *not* be used on anyone having pacemakers or other electronic devices inside their body. The human hand can be used instead because it's both magnetic and safe around the heart. My own preference is to use an *energy wand* so I don't have to be concerned with magnets.

If a practitioner is on the telephone or not physically present, then the magnet is of no concern when the practitioner moves the magnet over his own body *on behalf of* the client.

But how do we release Trapped Emotions? Let's find out.

These are the basic steps—*using muscle testing for most of them*—to release a Trapped Emotion in yourself related to a particular issue such as *right knee pain:*

1. Invoke divine guidance in whatever way is compatible with your beliefs, perhaps with a short prayer.

2. Determine by muscle testing if there is a Trapped Emotion that can be released which is contributing to your right knee pain. If no, stop.

3. If yes, use muscle testing to select the *exact* Trapped Emotion from a list of 60 Trapped Emotions in the book. It may be *personal* or *inherited* and you need to determine which by muscle testing.

4. Determine by muscle testing if you need to know any more information about the Trapped Emotion found.

5. If no, skip this step. If yes, use muscle testing to find any additional information *required* by the *body*. This may be the age when it was trapped, the location in your body and/or whose emotion it was if it was picked up from another person.

6. Release the Trapped Emotion with the *intent* to release it while amplifying that intention using any kind of magnet. Use your hand instead of a magnet if you have an implanted electrical device such as a pacemaker. Keep the magnet or your hand 1–2 inches away from your head

and move it along the g*overning meridian* from roughly the eyes to the nape of the neck. This is done 3 times if the Trapped Emotion is *personal* and 10 times if it is *inherited*.

7. Check with muscle testing to see if it has been released. If no, then repeat steps 5-7 until this Trapped Emotion is gone.

8. If yes, repeat steps 2–7 to release other Trapped Emotions until muscle testing indicates you're done.

The above steps are simplified. Please refer to *The Emotion Code* book to get detailed information needed in order to do this for yourself or for another. The book provides background information you *will* need to properly use the flowcharts.

The Emotion Code uses muscle testing to tap into the subconscious mind. Energy healers often refer to the subconscious mind as *the body* and I'll use that term from time to time. For example, if muscle testing indicates that our subconscious mind is willing to release a Trapped Emotion, we can also say that *the body* is willing to release a Trapped Emotion.

On any particular issue, it may take one or more sessions to clear Trapped Emotions outside or inside the Heart Wall because *the body* allows only a limited number of emotions to be cleared in any given session.

When *the body* is unwilling to let us remove any more Trapped Emotions for a given issue in that session, it may allow additional Trapped Emotions to be removed for a *different* problem in that same session.

Muscle testing will determine when no more Trapped Emotions can be removed for an issue or cleared from a Heart-Wall. More Trapped Emotions can often be removed later, perhaps in a few days.

Sometimes *the body* will allow only one or two Trapped Emotions to be released. If muscle testing indicates no Trapped Emotion can be released, then we ask, "Is there a *hidden* Trapped Emotion we can release now?" If yes, we proceed to release it without using the word *hidden* again for that particular Trapped Emotion. Many Trapped Emotions are hidden.

A practitioner can do Trapped Emotion clearing with you by telephone, via Skype or in person. It is also possible to do a long distance session for a client without being in voice communication.

I did an Emotion Code session on a lady in England, who granted me permission to do so. When I did the session, I did not talk with her as she was asleep in bed due to our time zone differences.

**Clearing a Heart-Wall**

As I've mentioned, Dr. Nelson has a flowchart in his book for clearing a Heart-Wall.

Clearing the Heart Wall for a child may take 1 session and an adult will often require 2–4 sessions (mine took 2 sessions). *The body* only allows a limited

*Expel an Emotion with a Refrigerator Magnet*

number of Heart-Wall emotions to be cleared in any particular session.

My wife Dorothy and I had an Emotion Code practitioner in another state perform several Emotion Code sessions on us. Dorothy's Heart-Wall, consisting of about 35 Trapped Emotions, was eliminated in 3 sessions of 30–60 minutes each.

Muscle testing determined that some of her Trapped Emotions were *personal*, originating in the womb or after birth. Others were *inherited* and one went back 7 generations. Our practitioner used the sway test to muscle test us. She stood while she was on the telephone with us.

After the Heart-Wall was cleared, Dorothy felt very relaxed and much more at peace and she had better color. The practitioner commented that Dorothy's voice had gotten stronger.

**Processing After an Emotion Code Session**

Following an Emotion Code session, you must adjust to the *surgical removal* of Trapped Emotions. About 80% of the time, there will be no visible symptoms. About 20% of the time, usually for no more than 1–2 days, you may feel more tired, which is common, feel out of sorts, have vivid dreams or experience emotional ups and downs. This is normal! You just need to drink lots of water, eat healthy food and get lots of rest so your body can heal itself.

I did a session for a young lady in another state by phone and found out, at the very end of the session, that she had been in tears the entire session. While that does not occur too often, it is a type of processing.

## Children and The Emotion Code

In *The Emotion Code* book, Dr. Nelson mentions a situation involving two of his own children who are fraternal twins. Let's call them twin A and twin B. Twin A was born first and twin B emerged 14 minutes later in critical condition and underwent a difficult first 10 days of life.

At about the age of four, twin A was speaking in sentences which twin B seemed unable to do. Twin B was also fearful and had claustrophobia. Dr. Nelson cleared a handful of Trapped Emotions and he said the next morning twin B was speaking in sentences like a little chatterbox. Dr. Nelson released these groups of Trapped Emotions:

1. **Panic.** Waiting in line to be born generated a Trapped Emotion of *panic*. This caused claustrophobia in twin B.

2. **Fear, abandonment and terror.** A few days after birth, his parents had been kicked out of his room at the hospital before the doctors did a spinal tap to give him antibiotics for a potentially deadly infection. Being deprived of his parents and having people stick needles into him, twin B screamed and generated Trapped Emotions of *fear*, *abandonment* and *terror*. This was a cause of his fear.

3. **Anger.** His Trapped Emotion of *anger* was inherited from a grandparent. This was the real problem with his reluctance to talk properly. Because of that inherited *anger* he felt he might hurt someone by speaking, so he resisted speaking in entire sentences.

**Animals and The Emotion Code**

What if you could help heal your pet?

It turns out that animals have very few Trapped Emotions—often a handful—as opposed to hundreds in the average man or woman. Animals, like humans, often get incredible results from The Emotion Code and they often occur much faster in animals.

The pet's owner or a practitioner, with permission of the owner, can use muscle testing to clear Trapped Emotions in the pet *without* touching the animal. A magnet can also be used on the animal directly but don't try that on a lion or a bear!

**Healing a Horse.** Dr. Nelson tells the story in his book of a horse that developed problems with its gait. Dr. Nelson found a Trapped Emotion of *sorrow*. Through muscle testing, he determined that the sorrow had something to do with a bird.

The owner then remembered that a baby bird had fallen out of its nest the week before and had died right in front of the horse. That created the Trapped Emotion of *sorrow*. After it was released by Dr. Nelson, the horse's gait returned to normal.

## Emotion Code Results

In *The Emotion Code* book, Dr. Nelson mentions perhaps 45 conditions where Trapped Emotions were the main or a contributing cause. Just a few of these issues are:

- Acid reflux, allergies, asthma, carpal tunnel,
- Crohn's Disease, depression, diabetes, dyslexia,
- fibromyalgia, heartburn, infertility, insomnia,
- joint, back, neck and other pain, lupus,
- learning disabilities, migraines, multiple sclerosis
- panic attacks, Parkinson's Disease, phobias,
- sinus problems, tennis elbow and vertigo.

As for myself, I have helped people with various problems. Let's now look at a few of the results I've seen when using The Emotion Code with clients.

**Shoulder Pain.** A friend with severe shoulder problems had a pain level of 9 on the 0–10 pain scale. He was undergoing physical therapy and was contemplating shoulder surgery. One Emotion Code session eliminated all his pain.

When he went to physical therapy a few days later he could do everything they requested—with no pain. Months later, he told me that his pain level had not exceeded a 1 since the only session we did together.

We did another session maybe a year later. He never did have surgery.

**Aggressive Dog.** A 10 year old dog had a fear of strangers and barked too much around them. It was a rescue dog and had been mistreated by a former owner who hit the dog with a broom at times. He was a puppy when the current owner got him.

I did the Emotion Code on that small but aggressive dog. It became very docile after one session in which Trapped Emotions, including some inherited ones, were released. This was done over the phone on an animal I'd never seen for an owner I'd never met in person and they both lived in another state. The owner was very pleased.

**Client Feedback after Heart-Wall Cleared.** After clearing a Heart-Wall, I received this email, shown as written, from the client who lived in another state:

> ... this healing process is HUGE within minutes. At the time I don't feel much different. It's very difficult to put into words. I want to say thanks again; this transformation was very unexpected. I wish I could understand how you do it, & know you're excellent at what ever you do. I think you understand more then I do. I can't wrap my brain around the experience. It's beyond words. I'm deeply grateful, & humbled.

## The Body Code

Dr. Nelson later developed another more comprehensive healing protocol called *The Body Code*. Like The Emotion Code, it uses muscle testing not only to help release Trapped Emotions but also to find and correct, in a variety of ways, many other imbalances in the body.

Imbalances have many causes, but Trapped Emotions are most often behind much of our physical and emotional pain and discomfort. A magnet is also used in The Body Code, along with intention, to release and correct many dozens or perhaps hundreds of different types of energetic problems in the body.

The Body Code is a form of energy work in which a practitioner, using muscle testing, identifies and corrects imbalances that can cause us emotional and physical problems. The human body has the powerful ability to heal itself—*if* conditions are right. The job of a Body Code practitioner is to improve those conditions.

Much of what is done using The Body Code involves releasing the energy of Trapped Emotions contributing to *emotional baggage*. When that happens, chakras and meridians are better balanced.

There is also a physical side where the practitioner looks for infections, toxins, nutritional and structural imbalances, then determines what is needed to restore balance in those areas. Many energetic and physical imbalances can be corrected immediately using

*Expel an Emotion with a Refrigerator Magnet*

magnets and intention.

In short, The Body Code is all about removing or correcting imbalances in order to make conditions right for the body to heal itself. It is not unusual for emotional or physical pain and discomfort to be reduced or eliminated in a single session or over a few sessions. Depending upon the issue, a number of sessions may be needed.

The Body Code, however, involves more ways of balancing the body than does The Emotion Code. An individual certified in The Body Code must first be certified in The Emotion Code. I received my certification in The Emotion Code in 2012 and in The Body Code in 2013.

A client sent me a testimonial email. She mentioned The Emotion Code which I had only used on her dog, her best buddy. This session was done long distance while we talked on the telephone.

I also performed some Body Code sessions on this client and her daughter. The Body Code includes The Emotion Code, although she only mentioned The Emotion Code in her email. Here is her email, shown pretty much *as is* although I changed spacing and a letter here and there for readability:

> John your sessions are awesome!!! They are working. Ever since you cracked my heart wall and introduced me to the emotion code my life has changed for the better. It really works!!! The sessions were short and I found that my

family responded right away. Even my best buddy is living the life I always dreamed of for him. My daughter is healthy and happy and I would advise the sessions to anyone who wants to live the life they always dreamed of. I can not imagine my life without having participated in these sessions.

**Emotion Code Advantages**

The Emotion Code can be done by telephone or in person. It's a simple procedure and it's possible to do it yourself using the flowcharts in The Emotion Code book, provided you have learned to muscle test yourself or know someone who can muscle test you.

It is not necessary to discuss *any* Trapped Emotion with a practitioner, so The Emotion Code or The Body Code is usually more relaxing for a client than traditional talk therapy.

**Emotion Code Limitations**

It may be difficult to muscle test yourself if you have tremors or physical disabilities. Magnets should not be used directly on people with pacemakers and other electrical devices in the body. However, as I mentioned, there are ways around this, such as by using the hand or an *energy wand*.

*Expel an Emotion with a Refrigerator Magnet*

# # #

See the *Resources Appendix* for more information about The Emotion Code. It will also show you how to find an Emotion Code practitioner who can work with you in person or long distance.

# Chapter Eight

## POINT YOUR FINGERS AT YOUR FACE TO HEAL

Imagine a healing art that seemingly came from God after more than a decade of prayer by a sincere man desperate to solve his wife's depression. Using it, her depression was gone in a few weeks.

How did this miracle healing method come about?

**Origin of Healing Codes**

Dr. Alexander Loyd is the primary author of *The Healing Code* book. His wife had suffered from clinical depression since their first year of marriage. He had a PhD in psychology, yet was unable to help her. They had tried everything—herbs, natural remedies, medication and more—with few results.

Twelve years into their marriage, Dr. Loyd was boarding an airplane to return home and was talking with his wife on the telephone. She was extremely distressed, so Dr. Loyd talked to her as long as he could, then boarded the plane. He prayed for an answer, as he had been doing for a dozen years.

This time, his prayers were answered and strange directions rushed into his mind as to what to do for his wife. The information came so quickly that he could barely write it down.

Once home, he used that knowledge with his wife whose depression was gone in about 45 minutes. Although the depression did eventually return, using the same procedures for about three more weeks caused her depression to disappear forever—and—she was able to give up all her medication.

This was done using a form of energy healing which involves setting an intention and pointing fingers at 4 special *healing centers* of the face and neck. We'll discuss all this a little later in this chapter. Dr. Loyd later named this method *The Healing Code,* a technique consisting of a small number of individual *Healing Codes.*

Dr. Loyd began sharing this technique with others. After a while, he had people reporting that multiple sclerosis, migraine headaches, cancer and other conditions had reversed themselves.

Dr. Loyd, who was an ordained minister, wanted to make sure that The Healing Code was in harmony with the Bible and could be shown effective using scientific and medical testing.

He determined that healing *issues of the heart,* which is what The Healing Code does, is completely compatible with biblical ideas—even more so than most healing methods.

Furthermore, he was able to find a scientific and accurate method of testing the stress that comes from unconscious, unhealed memories, beliefs and images buried in the spiritual *heart*. Using equipment to test Heart Rate Variability, the gold standard that tests stress of the autonomic nervous system, he was able to prove that The Healing Code lowers stress in the body. We've mentioned many times that decreasing stress leads to an improved immune system.

**Heart Issues and Stress**

Emotional stress suppresses the body's immune system. This is not only due to stress occurring today, but can also be due to stresses and traumas from childhood or even before birth. Stress is stored in cellular memory and is difficult to release by methods which focus on talking about the stressful situation.

Heart issues are emotional issues that are a constant source of stress for us. When we are guilty, ashamed, burdened, bitter, angry, frustrated or peeved, we are under stress.

We've already seen that just thinking about an emotional experience can trigger the *fight or flight* response and shut down our immune system.

Stress affects almost everybody. Dr. Loyd tells us that, when asked, 50% of people will state that they are stressed with an equal number saying they are not. However, scientific testing shows that's *not* true. In fact, some 95% of *all* people are stressed, despite what they believe.

# 6 LIFE CHANGING ENERGY HEALING METHODS

*The Healing Code* book tells how you can take an online test to show where you stand on various *issues of the heart*. Those issues are: unforgiveness, harmful actions, unhealthy beliefs, love, joy, peace, patience, kindness, goodness, trust, humility and self control.

## Unforgiveness and Disease

The word *unforgiveness* is not in the dictionary, but we know what it means. It is also the first *issue of the heart* mentioned in *The Healing Code* book.

Doctor Loyd and his co-author, Ben Johnson, MD, both tie cancer and serious diseases to emotional stress, specifically to unforgiveness. Dr. Loyd states in *The Healing Code* book:

> Unforgiveness is often betrayed by some form of anger or irritation or not wanting to be around a certain person. No matter what you call it, it can kill you.

Also in his book, Dr. Loyd mentions that the *Our Father* prayer actually mentions *forgiveness* twice. In it, Christians say:

> ...*forgive* us our trespasses as we *forgive* those who trespass against us ...

This prayer shows the importance of forgiveness. When we forgive others, we are also really healing *ourselves*. It is also important to forgive ourselves.

There's an old saying, with many variations, which goes like this: *holding onto anger is like drinking poison and expecting the other person to die.*

When we forgive, we are filling ourselves with love, the greatest healing force there is. As we've seen in the *Energy Healing* chapter, love has the highest frequency and is the ultimate healing force.

The *New Testament* says that *God is love* which is why billions of people use prayer as a form of *energy healing*. Larry Dossey, MD, wrote a book about the effectiveness of prayer, titled *Prayer is Good Medicine*. But not everyone is into prayer, love and peace.

Hatred and unforgiveness exist in this world, especially in Rwanda, where the Hutu government committed genocide on a much smaller ethnic group, the Tutsis, along with some moderate Hutus. Some 800,000 people were murdered. Forgiveness was in short supply as many families were decimated.

They say, "To err is human, to forgive, divine." While it is hard to forgive, some can forgive while others cannot. That happened in Rwanda after a Hutu man murdered the widowed mother of a Tutsi man named Ubald Rugirangoga.

Fr. Ubald is now a Catholic priest whom my wife and I've met when he visited Mississippi. For quite some time after his mother's murder, he couldn't sleep properly and wept at night. He felt despair since some 80 members of his family had been murdered.

Fr. Ubald eventually decided to forgive his mother's Hutu murderer who was then in prison. But he did not stop there. The murderer's wife had died, so Fr. Ubald paid the fees to educate the two children of his mother's murderer through high school, with plans to also pay their university fees.

Fr. Ubald now preaches everywhere on forgiveness and peace, especially in Rwanda, sometimes to an audience of 50,000 or more. He has also been a healing conduit for ill people and is fostering forgiveness throughout the world.

Now let's see how special Healing Code centers on the face and neck can help heal unforgiveness and other *issues of the heart* when we, unlike Fr. Ubald, seem unable to heal ourselves.

**Accessing Healing Code Centers**

The Healing Code involves examining an issue, saying a prayer expressing your intention for healing, then directing loving energy through the fingers into the body. The term Healing Codes refers to exactly which hands are pointed at which of four special locations on the face and neck, and in what sequence.

Behind these special locations on the head and neck are various glands, organs and parts of the brain and central nervous system. The positive energy entering these key centers will affect *every* cell, tissue, gland, organ and system of the body, resulting in stress reduction and a strengthened immune system.

These special control center locations are:

    1.   above the *bridge* of the nose, located between

the eyes and on the line connecting the eyebrows;

2. the *Adam's apple*;

3. the *jaw* area on the left and right side; and

4. the left and right *temples*.

The universal sequence in *The Healing Code* book directs you to point all your fingers and thumbs at each of these areas, one at a time. For simplicity, they are called *bridge, Adam's apple, jaw* and *temples*.

Fingers on both hands point to the bridge area for about 30 seconds, then to the Adam's apple for another 30 seconds. After that, the left hand points to the left jaw and the right hand to the right jaw, for about 30 seconds. Finally, the left hand points to the left temple and the right hand to the right temple, for about 30 seconds. This sequence is then repeated for 6–8 minutes. The entire session is performed 2–3 times each day.

The above one-size-fits-all generic Healing Codes are spelled out in Dr. Loyd's book. They will help anyone, but are not as specific to one's personal issues as are more *customized* codes, either from The Healing Codes Manual or that you receive from a certified Healing Codes Coach-Practitioner.

Later in this chapter, we'll see how this finger pointing is part of a typical Healing Code session. First, let's look into these specialized Healing Codes.

## Custom Healing Codes

For the universal Healing Codes, each hand points to the same area of the face or neck at the same time. For a particular issue, it is often more effective to point each hand at a different part of the face or neck and in different sequences, and to sometimes use more or less than the 4 sets of universal positions. For example, a 5 step sequence might be:

1. left hand—bridge, right hand—jaw; then

2. left hand—jaw, right hand—temple; then

3. both hands—Adam's apple; then

4. left hand—temple, right hand—jaw; then

5. both hands—bridge.

Healing Code practitioners can supply customized Healing Codes to clients for their particular *issue of the heart*. This is done using long distance energy field testing, a proprietary form of testing developed by Dr. Alex Loyd that Healing Code practitioners are trained to use. Using this special type of muscle testing, the practitioner determines the finger pointing sequence, the length of each session and the ideal total time spent over the day for all sessions.

After using Healing Codes for a period of time, perhaps a week or two, the client gets new codes from the practitioner for that issue or for another problem. After each period of time, the body changes and new Healing Codes will be more effective than the previous ones. The practitioner matches the custom Healing Code to the client's issue at a particular time and, as that issue heals, the energy shifts and the heart serves up what it is next ready to heal.

A practitioner can help you with all this by telephone, Skype or in person. Your practitioner only needs your voice frequency to get your custom Healing Code, so in-person consultation is not necessary, making it very convenient for both client and practitioner. You will do a customized Healing Code procedure several times a day on your own for perhaps 1–2 weeks. After that, a different set of customized codes can be made available to you, provided you have purchased additional sessions.

Some practitioners are also trained to do a *coach-guided code,* where they do Healing Codes *with you* over the phone. Some practitioners will record this and send it to you, as well as give you Healing Codes *to go* for your issue so you have a choice as to how to do it—listening to the recording or doing it on your own.

Doing a Healing Code with a practitioner can be especially powerful, as you have the combined power of more than one person, as well as the expert, loving guidance of the practitioner who is tuning in to your issue in real time.

Now we'll find out how Healing Codes reversed a so-called *incurable* disease.

**Healing Codes and ALS**

It was quite a shock to Ben Johnson, MD, a doctor who runs a center for alternative cancer treatments, when he was diagnosed with ALS (Lou Gehrig's Disease). Medical doctors believe that ALS is an *incurable* disease from which most die within 5 years.

After Dr. Johnson heard about The Healing Codes, he made contact with Dr. Loyd. Using custom Healing Code exercises from Dr. Loyd, Dr. Johnson reversed his ALS in less than 3 months. Later he co-authored The Healing Code book with Dr. Loyd. Be aware that Dr. Johnson did his custom Healing Codes for 30 minutes to 3 hours per day. He was desperate and determined to clear out every possible *heart issue* that could be contributing to his ALS.

In my opinion, their book has some of the most comprehensive and easy to read explanations of stress, the immune system and healing you will find. I've already mentioned that their book covers *issues of the heart*. We've already looked at one of them, namely *unforgiveness*.

Now let's take a brief look at how Healing Codes are used within a session. Lowering stress by healing *heart issues* can release pain, stress and illness. But what do we do to make that happen?

**A Healing Code Session**

A typical Healing Code session involves taking these steps which are laid out in far more detail in Dr. Loyd's book:

*Point Your Fingers at Your Face to Heal*

1. Rate an issue on the 0–10 pain scale.

2. Find unhealthy feelings or beliefs regarding your issue. In EFT, you may remember, we switch to the emotional stress *behind* the issue whenever there are no results working on a physical problem.

3. Look for earlier memories with the same feelings, rate them on the 0–10 pain scale, then pick the earliest or strongest one to work with.

4. Say the healing prayer of intention in *The Healing Code* book, modified to include your specific issue. We've already described the force of intention.

5. Point your fingers at the Healing Centers, as described earlier, using either the universal points from the book or custom points received from a Healing Code practitioner.

6. While doing the pointing, it's important to focus on something positive. You want the energy going from your fingertips to the Healing Centers to be positive. You can repeat a Truth Focus Statement (something your heart resonates with that you desire to become more true in your life), or simply think of a memory that fills you with love, joy or peace.

7. Rate your issue again on the 0–10 pain scale.

The Healing Code helped my wife Dorothy who received *customized* Healing Codes (not the universal ones in the book) through a Healing Code practitioner by telephone. The actual sessions were done several times that day and for a number of days afterward. When her codes *expired,* she got new ones.

After a number of weeks, Dorothy's color improved, her voice became stronger and her outlook on life was more optimistic.

**Healing Code Results**

*The Healing Code* book includes these and other conditions that have been reversed with Healing Codes:

- acid reflux, ALS (Lou Gehrig's Disease), cancer,
- chronic fatigue syndrome, chronic pain,
- closing a PFO (hole in heart), depression,
- emotional baggage, faulty beliefs, fibroid tumors,
- fibromyalgia, gallstones, hernia, leukemia,
- neurological disorders, night terrors, panic attacks,
- perfectionism, phobias, thyroid issues and vomiting.

**Healing Codes Advantages**

Healing Codes are easy to do, even by elementary school children who are able to read and point their fingers. The universal codes in *The Healing Code* book or manual can be done yourself with no assistance. You can also get customized Healing Codes from a practitioner by telephone.

It's possible to do the finger pointing mentally—in your mind—if it is too hard to hold up your fingers on or near your face. The book also tells how to do The Healing Code for another person, as I did for my wife, with her permission.

**Healing Codes Limitations**

Healing Codes take some time to do daily, ideally 3 times a day (40–60 minutes total per day). You need a practitioner to provide you with customized Healing Codes if you desire optimal results.

# # #

See the *Resources Appendix* for more information about Healing Codes. It will also show you how to find a Healing Code practitioner who can work with you in person or long distance.

# Chapter Nine

## READ AND REPAIR THE BODY'S LIGHT

Our body is full of light, called *biophotons*. Biophotons are weak light emitted by the cells of the body. Each one of our dozens of trillions of cells gives off up to 100,000 biophotons *every second*.

Photons are *information packets* determining how our cells communicate. They also control biochemical processes in the body and it is possible to use them to foster healing within us.

**Healing with Biophotons**

In the 1980s, Johan Boswinkel of the Netherlands translated an article from German to English. The article had been written by German physicist Fritz-Albert Popp, PhD, and was about biophotons, otherwise known as light, in the body.

Mr. Boswinkel, a man who had studied medicine, decided to see if he could read these biophotons, repair them, then put them back into the body. Mr. Boswinkel has been doing that for decades, correcting many chronic disease conditions. He and a team of people have helped over 100,000 people overcome many chronic illnesses.

Mr. Boswinkel studied Dr. Reinhard Voll, a German homeopathic physician who, in the mid-1900s, had developed an electronic machine which could measure information from acupuncture points located on the Chinese acupuncture meridians.

Mr. Boswinkel developed various machines to allow a practitioner to read, analyze and correct imbalances in a client's biophotons. The current and most advanced machine is called the *Chiren*.

The goal, like that of all energy healing, is to correct disturbances within the body so that the body can then heal itself. But first, we have to find the problems.

**Reading Biophotons**

These days, we hear about the speed of fiber optic cables which can control computers. Similarly, light controls biochemical processes throughout the body. By measuring the light photons, a biophoton therapist certified by Mr. Boswinkel, called a *biontologist,* can determine a bewildering amount of information about the body.

A biontologist can determine the condition of organs and glands, the presence of harmful pathogens, metals and toxins and can also detect problems with energy leaks and other imbalances.

Using the *Chiren*, the biontologist analyzes the

## Read and Repair the Body's Light

biophotons of the client. Two wires are connected to the *Chiren*. One of them is a grounding rod which the client holds in one hand while the biontologist touches various acupuncture points on the client's other hand using the pen-like probe at the end of the other wire.

The biontologist examines points on one of the client's hands, then repeats the process with the client's other hand. The *Chiren* emits a noise when the probe touches each point. The sound is either steady or it drops. Steady sounds indicate balanced points whereas *drops* indicate disturbances in the body associated with that acupuncture point.

My wife and I underwent biophoton therapy in California a few years ago. My biontologist, a young lady, started with my ring finger and then worked with other fingers. I'm a pattern person and asked her why she started with the middle of the hand instead of with the thumb or little finger. Her answer was that two critical hormonal system glands are examined using the ring finger: the pituitary gland and the parathyroid gland.

The *pituitary gland* at the base of the brain provides quality control for the body. If it is turned off, our body cannot distinguish between good guys and bad guys. Some energies, such as that from a polio vaccine, can disturb the pituitary gland, shutting it down. Biophoton therapy can turn it back on.

The *parathyroid gland* in the neck controls calcium in the body. This gland can be disturbed by tetanus or even by a tetanus shot which is a mild dose of tetanus.

According to Mr. Boswinkel, individuals with an unbalanced parathyroid gland may have Parkinson's disease or osteoporosis. Mr. Boswinkel has reversed Parkinson's disease when calcification in the body was not excessive.

When the examination of each hand is over, the biontologist then checks acupuncture points on one foot, then the other. The final result is a list of acupuncture points on the hands and feet which correspond with various organs, glands and systems within the body. Unbalanced points, those with *drops,* are flagged as problems.

The next step is for the biontologist to find a remedy which corrects each problem found.

**Repairing the Light**

Mr. Boswinkel determined that various frequencies, including those of homeopathic remedies, can be carried into the body along with biophotons. Let's briefly look at *homeopathy* which is based on the ancient Law of Similars. It originated with Hippocrates, the *Father of Medicine,* who believed that a substance that can *cause* a problem is also able to *cure* that same condition.

Most readers are vaguely familiar with homeopathic medicine. These days, you can find homeopathic eyedrops and other homeopathic medicines in local stores. They usually look like water and for good reason—they are mostly water.

Water has the property of *memory*. In other words, any energy that comes in contact with water can be stored, somehow, *inside* the water. In homeopathy, water is added to a beneficial substance, usually something *akin to* some health issue, because the principle of homeopathy is that *like cures like*. This solution is then diluted over and over and over again.

In cases of extreme dilution, the best chemist in the world cannot find *any* of the original substance in the water. This is one of the reasons why homeopathy is considered very safe.

A late friend of mine, a well known Hollywood actor, was trying to import a rattlesnake venom homeopathic solution into the United States from a foreign country. The United States government told him that it didn't contain any rattlesnake venom so he couldn't import it. Someone in the government did not realize that homeopathic solutions are often diluted to the point where the original substance cannot be detected.

That's enough about homeopathy. But how are suitable healing frequencies chosen by the biontologist? The *Chiren* is a computer which contains numerous healing frequencies. The biontologist uses the *Chiren* to select the appropriate remedy for each energy imbalance detected. For example, the frequencies of intestinal flora, the friendly bacteria in probiotics, are sometimes used to correct intestinal problems.

After the problems have been identified in the client's energy system and corrective remedial frequencies have been chosen, the biontologist uses the *Chiren* to read biophotons from one of the client's hands. The *Chiren* alters them in these 3 ways:

1. The *good* light, the coherent light, is amplified to strengthen it.

2. The incoherent or chaotic *bad* light, is changed so that it is canceled out, much like noise canceling headphones eliminate background noise.

3. Homeopathic or other beneficial frequencies are added to the biophotons. These can assist the body in detoxifying itself, for example, by strengthening the liver or kidneys. Other frequencies can help circulation, support the adrenal glands and provide emotional support.

The biophotons read using one hand are modified inside the *Chiren*, then sent into the other hand for perhaps 10 minutes. When that hand is finished, the same thing is done with the feet on a footplate, using a different set of remedies.

## Checking Results

After putting the corrected light into the hands and feet, the biontologist rechecks points on the hands and feet that were unbalanced. Ideally, each point initially showing a *drop* should now be balanced. Over time, each point may stay balanced or it may revert to an unbalanced state. In my experience, *drops* are

*Read and Repair the Body's Light*

rarely found during this re-checking of points.

The biontologist can look at charts of the hands and feet and see improvements over time. Since the body changes often, something that is currently balanced may become unbalanced later on. For example, if you get food poisoning, then that imbalance will show up if you have a biophoton treatment around that time.

**Biophoton Therapy Effectiveness**

Mr. Boswinkel has been doing biophoton therapy for some 30 years, so his expertise is amazing and unique. A few years ago, he stated that his personal reversal rate for all chronic diseases was 93% and that of his worldwide practitioners was about 80%.

Mr. Boswinkel knows that when the body becomes balanced using biophotons and healing frequencies, it can begin to reverse disease, pain and discomfort caused by disruptive energy. He applies this same methodology to *any* disease, whether it be cancer or any other illness.

Balancing the pituitary gland is most important since it must be functioning properly to identify *bad guys* and allow our immune system to destroy them.

In Traditional Chinese Medicine, organs are paired. The liver is paired with the gallbladder. With coupled organs, when one is disturbed, so often is the other. The liver is associated with muscle strength and the gallbladder with muscle tension.

So, muscle weakness is often related to liver

imbalances and muscle spasms are connected to gallbladder problems. Diseases like Parkinson's and epilepsy may be due, in part, to imbalances in these organs.

One biontologist had a client, a young lady in her 20s, with a history of epileptic seizures which had been occurring several times each week during her entire life. The client informed the biontologist that she had not had a seizure during the entire two weeks following her second session. She had never gone that long without a seizure in her life.

A friend of mine had hearing problems, especially with his left ear. He had a biophoton treatment and, a few days later, he was able to hear with a cell phone up to his left ear, something he could not do before his treatment.

The suggested treatment for any illness is at least 3 treatments about a week apart. The body detoxifies for about 3 days following a treatment and a day of rest is then needed, so a client usually waits 5–7 days minimum between treatments. Some serious diseases might require even 20 or more treatments.

The *Chiren* also has special modes to treat whiplash and scar tissue. At my first treatment, my biontologist treated me for both whiplash and several scars.

### Long Distance and Animal Therapy

My wife and I have successfully done many *long distance* biophoton therapy treatments with a lady in the Netherlands, nearly 5,000 miles away. We use

Skype to talk with our biontologist.

Taking long distance measurements with the *Chiren* is done using a human *surrogate* connected to the *Chiren*. Our Dutch biontologist has acted as the surrogate for my wife and also for myself. Since biophoton therapy can be done on every living creature, she often does the same for an animal. Long distance *treatment* is done using a picture of the human or animal.

Most biontologists only do treatments in person as long distance sessions are taught, but not stressed, in their basic training. A few biontologists with advanced training do long distance sessions. Our biontologist did the treatment of my wife using a photograph of my wife. It appears impossible to many, but it works.

Our European biontologist once worked on a horse that was not able to conceive. Her testing found bacteria in the horse that was causing the problem. After treatment, the horse ended up with a much sweeter disposition and was able to easily get pregnant. It only took two biophoton sessions.

**Biophoton Results**

Since biophoton therapy balances the entire body it can, in theory, improve any condition in the body. It has been shown effective with numerous health issues. Just a few conditions reversed or made better with biophoton therapy include:

- ADHD, adrenal fatigue, asthma, candida,

- cardiovascular, depression, dyslexia, epilepsy,
- fibroid tumors, food allergies, frozen shoulders,
- glaucoma, hearing problems, hormonal imbalances,
- infections, intestinal issues, lack of mental focus,
- low energy, lupus, migraine headaches,
- Parkinson's Disease, physical pain, PTSD,
- scar shrinking, skin problems, sleep problems,
- stress, thyroid problems, tumors and whiplash.

**Biophoton Therapy Advantages**

Biophoton therapy is non-invasive, with nothing entering the body except one's own modified light, plus some beneficial homeopathic or other frequencies. This therapy does not weaken the immune system or vital organs as do most medicines, surgery and radiation.

Mr. Boswinkel resides in the Netherlands, but there are other biontologists who may be able to work on you. As I've mentioned, my wife and I underwent biophoton therapy in California in person. But, since we live in Mississippi, we later opted for long distance sessions with a lady in the Netherlands.

## Biophoton Therapy Limitations

For some unknown reason, persons taking proton inhibitors and men who have had a vasectomy are sometimes resistant to biophoton therapy. Some other clients, however, have more serious biophoton treatment problems, as we'll now see.

Mr. Boswinkel once treated a client who had a transplanted kidney. The client's other kidney was not working. After treatment, there was good news and bad news.

The bad news was that the client's body began rejecting the transplanted kidney because the therapy had woken up the pituitary gland whose job, among others, is to reject *foreign* substances in the body. These strangers can be harmful bacteria or, in this case, the kidney originally belonging to another person.

The good news is that the treatment also woke up the client's dormant kidney. As a result of this incident, clients are no longer accepted for treatment who have had organ transplants or who have animal parts, such as pig valves, in their body.

Lastly, only a few biontologists do long distance sessions.

# # #

See the *Resources Appendix* for more information about biophoton therapy. It will also show you how to find a biontologist who can perform biophoton therapy with the *Chiren*.

# Chapter Ten

## USE A LITTLE KNOWN SYSTEM OF THE BODY TO HEAL

Imagine stress and trauma being treated without any type of talk therapy while you are lying down. A therapist listens to a system of the body which is not found in most medical books, then makes gentle corrections to your body when that system is not flowing properly.

The system missing from most medical books is the *craniosacral system*.

### The Craniosacral System

The craniosacral system was discovered in the United States by Dr. John Upledger in 1972. While he was assisting a surgeon who was performing neck surgery, Dr. Upledger first noticed the movement of the *dura mater* which he subsequently investigated over many decades.

The word craniosacral is composed of two parts. The first part, *cranio,* refers to the cranium—the part of the skull which is the container for the brain. The second part, *sacral,* refers to the sacrum—the bottom of the spinal column or tailbone. Craniosacral refers to the portion of the body which includes the skull and spine.

We learn in school about systems in the body. They include the circulatory system, muscular system, lymphatic system, digestive system and others. Most medical books fail to mention the craniosacral system as a bodily system, even though it has been known for decades.

It is comprised of these two parts:

1. **The *dura mater*.** This is a waterproof bag or sack, the outer layer of a three layered membrane which we know as the *meninges*. It also serves as a liner for the *cranium* and contains the brain and spinal cord. It also contains two glands inside the head: the pituitary master gland and the pineal gland.

2. **The craniosacral fluid.** This fluid is inside the *dura mater*.

Dr. Sutherland discovered that the craniosacral fluid is like the tide: it rolls in and rolls out, approximately 8–12 times a minute. Even though the craniosacral fluid encloses the brain and spine, this *tide* can be felt throughout the entire body.

When the craniosacral tide is weak, we're not healthy. When the tide is out of balance, for example, between our right and left hips, this indicates a problem in the body.

Palpitating or feeling the tide is most important in Craniosacral Therapy.

## Craniosacral Therapy (CST)

Craniosacral Therapy was developed in the 1970s by an osteopathic physician, Dr. John E. Upledger, at Michigan State University. It is partially based on discoveries in the area of cranial osteopathy made decades earlier by osteopath William Garner Sutherland.

Craniosacral Therapy is an extremely gentle healing art in which a practitioner monitors, using gentle touch, the rhythm of the craniosacral system. The therapist exerts a feeling pressure of approximately 5 grams or less on adults, about the weight of a nickel, and about 1 gram or less for infants.

The client is usually lying down, face up and fully clothed in comfortable clothing on a massage table.

The therapist evaluates restrictions, obstructions and other imbalances in the movement of the cerebrospinal fluid then, using *intuition*, gently *moves energy*. These energetic adjustments put the body into a more balanced state, often eliminating stress and trauma, resulting in a stronger immune system.

Some clients, such as myself, fall asleep during a session. My treatment sessions often last close to two hours, but those of some therapists may last an hour or less. Some clients *re-live* emotional trauma as it is released.

After a session, some clients are very tired while others are energized. The body heals itself and the therapy puts the healing systems of the body in a more effective state to do so. Results can take place quickly or over days or weeks.

**Craniosacral Therapy Results**

Craniosacral Therapy has helped people of all ages, from newborn infants to very senior citizens. My mom uses Craniosacral Therapy and that is perhaps one reason she has now passed the age of 100.

Craniosacral Therapy balances the body and enables the immune system, the body's healing system, to do its job and help heal the body. Since disease is due to a compromised immune system, Craniosacral Therapy has helped correct many types of problems, including:

- arthritis, autism, brain trauma,
- bruxism (teeth grinding), chronic pain, coma,
- depression, ear and eye problems, fibromyalgia,
- hyperactivity, headaches (including migraines),
- injuries, learning disabilities,
- physical and emotional trauma, PTSD,
- post surgical issues, rheumatoid arthritis,

*Use a Little Known System of the Body to Heal*

- scoliosis, spinal injuries, stress, stroke, tension,
- TMJ (jaw problems), vertigo and whiplash.

One of the reasons for this is that the craniosacral system touches the *entire* body directly or indirectly. It directly surrounds the brain and spine, including their bones.

Bones, even those in the head, are mobile. They can be coaxed back into their correct positions by a skilled therapist. This is valuable for those, like my wife, who have suffered whiplash. It is highly beneficial for anyone with a brain injury.

Furthermore, since the central nervous system is affected by bones in the head and spine, the health of the entire body can often be improved by a craniosacral therapist who affects, although sometimes indirectly, the central nervous system.

Many Craniosacral Therapy stories are mentioned in Dr. John Upledger's book titled *Your Inner Physician and You* and others are mentioned on the website of the Upledger Institute.

Dr. Upledger believed that 80–85% of headaches respond favorably to Craniosacral Therapy. He was also of the opinion that about half of all headache problems could be traced back to a blow to the tailbone that had happened perhaps months or years before.

Let's now examine stress and trauma in light of

Craniosacral Therapy.

**Releasing Energy Cysts and Emotions**

When the body is subjected to a blow, the energy travels through the body until it can go no further. This traumatic energy is then confined to that part of the body, perhaps the pelvis or a hip where the injury energy becomes a very small ball of energy which Dr. Upledger named an *energy cyst*.

The rest of the body expends valuable energy resources in trying to compensate for the distortion caused by the energy cyst. Eventually, even decades later, the body becomes less and less able to adjust to the energy cyst and we start noticing symptoms such as discomfort and pain.

As for emotions, we've already seen that lodged or embedded emotions are often between the size of an orange and that of a grapefruit. They can—and do—affect the tissues around them.

Craniosacral Therapy uses an advanced technique, developed by Dr. Upledger, called SomatoEmotional Release (SER). During SomatoEmotional Release, the therapist uses the craniosacral rhythm as well as a combination of touch, intuition and moving energy to defuse energy cysts and also to release the energy associated with an emotion stuck in the body. This unique procedure allows the body to heal.

**Disoriented Diver**

Mary Ellen Clark won a bronze medal in 10 Meter

*Use a Little Known System of the Body to Heal*

Platform Diving in the Summer Olympics in Barcelona in 1992. A few years later, she developed vertigo and was only able to train sporadically as a diver.

You see, it's difficult to be a diver when vertigo sometimes causes you to try to swim to the *bottom* of the pool after a dive. She tried training for a while with divers on the side of the pool to help her if she swam down instead of up. In January of 1995, she was forced to give up diving.

She tried everything she could to correct her problem —the Mayo Clinic, acupuncture, medication, herbs and many therapies. Nobody could correct her vertigo. She even found a few divers around the world with vertigo but learned that *none* of them had ever returned to diving.

In September of 1995, about a year before the Atlanta Summer Olympics, she turned to Dr. Upledger and Craniosacral Therapy for help. She was not disappointed.

Dr. Upledger eliminated several energy cysts, corrected a knee previously injured on a trampoline, adjusted her spine and pelvis, as well as performing various other Craniosacral Therapy techniques.

Craniosacral Therapy gave her the opportunity to resume diving—without vertigo—in the next few months. At the age of 33, which is considered old for a competitive diver, Mary Ellen Clark won her second straight diving bronze medal at the 1996 Atlanta

Summer Olympics!

**Veterans and PTSD**

Post Traumatic Stress Disorder (PTSD) upsets the lives of veterans and others, both in the daytime and at night. People with PTSD often have trouble sleeping and suffer from panic attacks, lack of concentration, violent episodes, nightmares, sweating, paranoia, depression, addictions as well as from many other debilitating health issues.

The key to ameliorating PTSD symptoms with Craniosacral Therapy is releasing traumatic energy from the body. Many individual craniosacral therapists, such as mine, have had tremendous success treating people with PTSD. Furthermore, the Upledger Institute in Florida has a special program for people with PTSD.

Dr. Upledger once conducted a special two-week intensive program for 6 veterans suffering from PTSD. This PTSD healing exercise involved 18 therapists. The veterans spent most of each day in treatment along with their therapists.

Three years later:

- 4 veterans were gainfully employed and were doing very well in life.

- 1 veteran, who had experienced excellent results, had died in an auto accident after deciding to train in Craniosacral Therapy to work with other veterans suffering from PTSD.

- 1 veteran was having occasional bouts with alcohol, an *improvement* in this individual's life because he was no longer using hard drugs as he had been doing prior to Craniosacral Therapy. Furthermore, this individual had attempted suicide three times prior to Craniosacral Therapy, but not once afterward.

**Intensive CST Programs**

The Upledger Institute lists these 9 special intensive programs on their website:

1. Concussion Program
2. Post Traumatic Stress Disorder Relief
3. Dolphin Assisted Therapy
4. Brain & Spinal Cord Dysfunction
5. Learning Disabilities in Children
6. Autism
7. Addictive Behaviors
8. Grief and Depression
9. Therapist Rejuvenation

Now let's look at one of these programs in which human therapists are aided by dolphins.

## Dolphins Heal Humans

In 1996, Dr. Upledger started a program in Florida involving dolphins. The Upledger Institute today has a program of using wild dolphins to heal clients. This program is currently conducted in the Bahamas where a client spends time in the ocean with several therapists and the *wild* dolphins that show up to help out.

Dr. Upledger believed that dolphins somehow sense what kind of energy is needed by a given patient. They then produce the appropriate beneficial high frequency healing sounds.

In his book, Dr. Upledger describes a session in which he, assisted by two other therapists, were in the ocean treating a client with a misaligned pelvis. Several wild dolphins came up behind the therapists and put their snouts, called rostrums, in the back of the therapists, but did *not* touch the client.

Since the therapists were touching the patient, the energy emitted by each dolphin got transferred to the client. When this happened, Dr. Upledger was able to feel the release of the patient's pelvis.

The result was astounding. Before entering the water, the patient's right leg was about 3 inches longer then the left leg. After the dolphin-assisted treatment, the difference between the legs was 1 inch.

What is interesting about this treatment is that the dolphins are wild and have never attended medical school. Despite that, wild dolphins have helped many patients get better—without even being on the payroll of the Upledger Institute!

## Craniosacral Therapy Advantages

Craniosacral Therapy is a gentle healing art which treats the whole body, correcting physical and energetic imbalances found by the therapist. It restores harmony within the body and a therapist can even adjust bones in the head which are out of position due to trauma or other reasons.

A skilled craniosacral therapist can find and gently reverse many emotionally stressful and traumatic conditions and other imbalances which often contribute to vertigo, headaches, Traumatic Brain Injury (TBI), whiplash, PTSD and many other health issues.

## Craniosacral Therapy Limitations

Practitioners of Craniosacral Therapy vary in skill, so it is often preferable, but sometimes difficult, to find a very experienced and knowledgeable therapist close to where you live. Therapists are listed on the Upledger Institute website. Persons with acute aneurysms, cerebral hemorrhage and bleeding in the head should normally not use Craniosacral Therapy.

# # #

See the *Resources Appendix* for more information about Craniosacral Therapy. It will also show you how to find a craniosacral therapist.

# Chapter Eleven

## OXYGENATE YOUR BLOOD IN MINUTES LYING DOWN

Imagine a medical device you can buy and use at home for the cost of a small computer and that has a positive effect on dozens or hundreds of medical conditions involving pain, stress, discomfort and illness.

Does this sound like fantasy? I assure you it's real. This miraculous product is the Original Chi Machine, invented by a doctor. It's used in some Japanese hospitals and is a medical device in various countries.

**The Chi Machine**

One day, I heard a lady named Jo being interviewed on the radio about a medical device called a *Chi Machine*. She told how this machine was invented, what it did, and how it had greatly helped her family.

Jo mentioned that Dr. Shizuo Inoue, a medical doctor in Japan, was watching goldfish swim in the early 1960s. He noticed the movement of their tails, back and forth and slightly up and down, like a figure eight on its side. He theorized that this goldfish motion was somehow connected with how fish get oxygen.

Some time later, Dr. Inoue was in a train station when a man collapsed and was dying. Dr. Inoue grabbed the man's ankles, raised his legs, and made the *goldfish motion* with the man's feet, for about 30 minutes, thus saving the man's life. He also did this on another occasion for another individual.

Dr. Inoue then invented a machine, the first Chi Machine, that simulated the motion of the tail of the goldfish. The Chi Machine was tested with the help of over 100,000 people. This device, sometimes called the Original Chi Machine, is now marketed worldwide and has been available in the United States for well over a decade.

Jo said that she had bought her Chi Machine sight unseen in the hope that it might help her acute condition of achy legs and purple toes—and it did.

She then tried it out on her mother who could not drive after having a brain tumor the size of a baseball removed. She also had congestive heart failure and had lost the use of 1–1/2 lungs due to blood clots following her brain surgery.

The Chi Machine miraculously healed her mother's brain, eliminated her congestive heart failure, helped her regain full use of *both* lungs—and—get her drivers license again. I was captivated.

By the way, the first time I met Jo's mom was after she'd driven, by herself, from eastern Mississippi to Covington, Louisiana, about a 3 hour drive. This was a

*Oxygenate Your Blood in Minutes Lying Down*

lady who used to sit all day long in a chair a few years earlier with almost no quality of life.

Back to the Chi Machine. I was very used to the concept of *chi*—the Chinese word for energy or life force—because I'd been doing *tai chi* for some years and had felt *chi* in my body many times.

I contacted Jo in Louisiana and she loaned me a Chi Machine even though I, like some of her family, lived in Mississippi.

**My Initial Chi Machine Experience**

Jo demonstrated the Chi Machine for me and I liked it. My wife also thought it was good. Some people can feel *chi* energy when the machine is moving and others feel a rush of *chi* after it stops. Much of the benefit takes place over the next few minutes after the machine stops.

I felt nothing special but my wife, when the machine stopped, felt an intense rush of energy from her feet to her head. She said, "That's the most electricity I've felt since I put my hand in a defective toaster!"

Jo gave me permission to loan it to a friend of mine. He was a smoker with breathing problems.

I showed him and his wife how to use the machine and these 4 amazing stories emerged:

1. He used the Chi Machine for 3–5 minutes. His wife told me that while he was on the Chi Machine, she noticed that he was *breathing*

*better than he had in a long time.* He also felt so much better in many ways.

2. His wife, who had had back surgery about a year and a half earlier, told me that, after a few days on the Chi Machine, *she had never felt better in her life.*

3. A few days later, she told me how the Chi Machine helped their daughter. Their daughter, who had had neck surgery about a year earlier, experienced headaches every waking moment. *After 5 minutes on the Chi Machine, she was able to remain free of headaches for about 24 hours.* Their daughter lived in another city so was not able to use it often. However, whenever she used the Chi Machine, her headaches stopped for about a day after each use.

4. A day or two later, their daughter's boyfriend tried the Chi Machine for about 6 minutes one morning. He was a diabetic, who had lost feeling in his feet, a condition called neuropathy. That night he stepped on something—*and felt it*—for the first time in many months.

Seeing all these benefits from the Chi Machine, *all within one week*, I bought a Chi Machine, became a distributor and have never regretted it.

My own health improved and I needed about 30 minutes less sleep per night when using the Chi Machine just before bedtime. We then bought a Chi

Machine for my mother who was then 87.

My mom also had some nice results. The Chi Machine eliminated tiredness in her legs and helped to alleviate her problems with arthritis, constipation and circulation. It also helped her back and neck and partially eliminated the scoliosis in her spine.

**Benefits of the Original Chi Machine**

These 6 benefits are mentioned in the Canadian Original Chi Machine brochure, along with my own comments and observations:

1. **Cellular Activation.** The Chi Machine causes the bronchioles in the lungs to open up and allow more oxygen in the air in our lungs to enter the bloodstream. The motion of the machine also causes the lymph system to move, picking up the oxygen from the bloodstream and transporting it the rest of the way to where it is needed by each cell. This results in an activated and more efficient cell.

2. **Spinal Balancing.** You use the Chi Machine lying down, with *no weight* on the spine. Misalignment of spinal disks is often corrected and, since nerves pass through the spinal bones, pinched nerves are often released. People with back and neck problems often see relief.

3. **Improving the Immune System.** The Chi Machine causes an increase in globulin which boosts the immune system, enabling the body

to better fight disease.

4. **Blood Production.** There is an increased production of blood in the bone marrow of the spine.

5. **Restoration of Balance to the Autonomic Nervous System.** This helps the body relax, reducing stress.

6. **Exercising Internal Organs.** The *chi* life force energy to each organ is improved. The energy in the acupuncture meridians and in the chakras are much improved. This has been verified with kirlian photography, a technique of photographing energy. *Qigong* masters also attest that *chi* is indeed flowing within the body while using the machine and afterward.

You can see from the above that the Chi Machine seems to help just about every part of the body. But what do medical doctors say?

Nathaniel Lipton, MD, compiled a book in 2004 titled *The Collection*. It consists of about 200 testimonials from people using the Chi Machine.

His testimonials fall into about 35 different categories. Some of them are:

- allergies, asthma, arthritis, back and other pain,

- depression, dermatitis, diabetes, dyslexia,

- fibromyalgia, headache, insomnia, lupus,
- multiple sclerosis, neuropathy, paralysis,
- Parkinson's Disease, scoliosis, stress,
- swollen ankles, stroke, trauma and weight loss.

Some testimonials were about complete recovery and others described various levels of positive results. Since the Chi Machine improves oxygen and energy within the body, it's no wonder so many conditions were improved.

In the front of his book, Dr. Lipton lists these 12 commonly reported benefits of the Chi Machine:

1. Relief from muscle stiffness and chronic pain—especially back and neck pain;
2. Improved blood circulation;
3. Improved lymphatic drainage;
4. Improved function of the internal organs;
5. Stronger immune system;
6. Relief from headaches;
7. More energy and greater sense of well-being;
8. Stronger and more limber spine and joints;
9. Better skin tone;

10. Sounder more restful sleep;

11. Weight loss, firming and toning of the thighs, hips, buttocks and breasts; and

12. Greatly increased ability to relax and let go of stress and tension.

**Oxygen and the Chi Machine**

We saw in the *Emotional Stress Sabotages Health* chapter that Nobel Prize winner Dr. Otto Warburg linked cancer to lack of oxygen and that doctors have associated oxygen deficiency with most diseases.

The Chi Machine is sometimes called an *Aerobic Exerciser*. In Japanese, the Chi Machine is called a *Goldfish Exercise Machine*. Aerobic exercise gives us more oxygen, so the Chi Machine is truly an aerobic exercise machine.

The Canadian Original Chi Machine Brochure, under a section called Whole Body Massage, says this:

> A full body massage, including internal organs and all body systems, occurs with the massager's use. A fifteen minute massage is estimated to be the equivalent of walking ten thousand paces (about 90 minutes) in terms of body oxygenation.

Wow! Just fifteen minutes on the Chi Machine gives you as much extra oxygen as you'd get if you went outside and walked for an hour and a half.

Dr. Inoue, the inventor of the Chi Machine, was a famous doctor who:

1. was president of the Oxygen Health Association;

2. was director of Japan's Health Association;

3. studied the effects of oxygen on the body for 38 years;

4. believed that insufficient oxygen was a *cause* of illness and that oxygen was a *solution* to disease; and

5. received a patent for his Chi Machine about 1990, after testing it on some 100,000 individuals. His international patents preclude anyone from copying the machine's distinct, well tested parameters. This means that any *knockoff* machine, whatever the price, is *not compatible with the human body* and that can be proven via muscle testing.

Ed McCabe, the most famous oxygen therapy journalist in the world, discusses the Chi Machine several times in his book, *Flood Your Body with Oxygen*. Mr. McCabe touts its ability to oxygenate the body and remove toxins by activating the lymph system. He even has several pictures of the Chi Machine in his book.

## The Chi Machine Alters Blood in Minutes

A lady named Kathryn Shaw took 3 blood samples from several people:

1. before they got on the Chi machine;

2. after using the Chi Machine for 3 minutes; and

3. after a total of 13 minutes on the Chi Machine.

Before getting on the Chi Machine, some of the people had clumped up blood—called *rouleaux* blood—which does not carry much oxygen to the cells. How did she know this? She examined all the blood samples under a dark field microscope.

After 3 minutes on the Chi machine, the blood for all participants showed their red blood cells were largely separated, one from another, although they were not yet moving rapidly.

After 13 minutes on the Chi machine, the microscope showed that the blood of *all* subjects was flowing very well and that red blood cells were not touching each other. This means the red blood cells are able to allow more oxygen molecules to attach to the hemoglobin sites on the red blood cells.

So, if you want more oxygen in your blood and cells, you can simply use the Chi Machine for a few minutes or, ideally, perhaps 10 to 15 minutes or even longer. Remember, 15 minutes on the Chi Machine gives you the amount of oxygen you would get if you went out and walked for an hour and a half.

**The Chi Machine Boosts the Body's Energy**

A chiropractor, Dr. David Moths, had a company take 4 special photographs of his *aura*:

1. before he used the Chi Machine;

2. after 10 minutes on the Chi Machine;

3. after 15 minutes on the Chi Machine; and

4. after 20 minutes on the Chi Machine.

The aura and different chakras of the body showed up in various colors. At 15 minutes the body was much more vibrant than before using the Chi Machine. However, at 20 minutes there was a huge increase in the intensity of the energy in the chakras.

For this reason, I often use the Chi Machine for 30 minutes, which is equivalent to the amount of extra oxygen I'd get if I walked for 3 hours!

My mom, who is over 100 years old, also regularly uses the Chi Machine for 20–30 minutes at a time. She even used it on her hundredth birthday.

**How to Use the Chi Machine**

The most important steps in using the Chi Machine are:

1. Drink some water—it lets *chi* flow more easily.

2. Lie down with your feet on the machine, with no pillow, although the neck and knees can be supported if needed.

3. Set the Chi Machine timer for 3–5 minutes if you have never used it before. You will enter a deeper brain wave state. It is possible to fall asleep when the machine is moving and especially after it stops.

4. When the machine stops, you stay motionless for several minutes. I set a timer before I start the machine to go off about 3 minutes *after* the machine stops. Much of the work is being done in those few extra minutes.

5. You can then do, if you like, a standard spine stretching exercise. This optional exercise is performed while lying on your back, with your feet on the ground close to your bottom, your knees in the air and your arms out to the side, palms up. You then *gently* turn your head to the right and knees to the left, then hold for a few seconds. You then switch directions and repeat several times. When I first started using the Chi Machine I'd hear bones moving and cracking in my low back as I did this exercise because the Chi Machine had loosened them up.

6. *Slowly* get up as a very small number of people may feel a bit woozy. This is rare, but it can happen.

7. Drink some more water—to help remove toxins because oxygen detoxifies the body.

Please be aware that if you're using the Chi Machine at night before going to bed, get ready for bed *before* using the machine. After using the machine, drink some water, use the toilet if needed, then go immediately to bed. But, if you decide to watch television, then the oxygen will kick in and you may end up *wide awake* instead of remaining in the deeper brain wave state you were in while you were on the machine.

**Chi Machine Advantages**

The Sun Ancon Original Chi Machine, distributed worldwide outside of Japan by Hsin Ten Enterprises (HTE), is easy to use and provides a way to exercise without weight on the spine. It's not a toy but it is a Class 1 medical device in the United States, regulated by the Food and Drug Administration (FDA). It is also a medical device in Canada.

In Japan, it's a medical device used in various hospitals. The Chi Machine is a one-time expense, costing about the same as an inexpensive computer.

**Chi Machine Limitations**

The Chi Machine is hard to use if you cannot lie down on the floor. However, it can be used on a firm bed provided it sits on a hard surface—like a large wooden cutting board—to allow cooling under the machine.

There are some people who should probably not use it: those with broken bones or recovering from bone and other surgeries. There used to be a caution for pregnant women, but many doctors believe that the

Chi Machine should be used during most or all of pregnancy.

Once again, *check with your doctor* if you have any doubts about using it safely. People with extremely serious conditions have sometimes begun using it for 1 minute or less.

# # #

See the *Resources Appendix* for more information about The Chi Machine. It will also show you how to purchase the Original Chi Machine which you can use in your own home.

# Final Thoughts

This book was about *good guys* and *bad guys* with regard to our health. My goal was to show you ways of eradicating some of the enemies.

The heroes are *oxygen* and our *immune system*. Oxygen provides fuel or power for our cells and lack of it causes cancer and almost every other illness. Our immune system is our protection, much like a police or fire department. It guards our cells from bacteria, viruses and more, keeping us healthy.

All healthy practices and healing modalities should increase our oxygen and boost our immune system. When we're healthy and well oxygenated, our cellular environment is slightly alkaline and our overall body frequency is high.

The villains are many types of *stressors*. In this book we've concentrated on these destructive ones: mental and physical trauma, faulty and negative thoughts, as well as stress and harmful emotions. Stress and emotional baggage impact the health of our body, mind and spirit.

Emotions can be good or bad, healthy or damaging. Health improves when we reduce our negative thoughts and emotions and increase our positive ones, especially high frequency love.

Trauma affects the brain and organs of the body, triggering cancer and many diseases. Healing a disease ideally means removing the *cause* of the disease, which is most often stress or trauma.

But, up until now, there haven't been very many good ways to get rid of emotional toxins, emotional stress, emotional baggage—whatever name we give it. But, that's why I wrote this book for you—to make you aware of some very powerful stress eliminating techniques.

Mainstream medicine has difficulty addressing emotional stress apart from traditional talk therapy that can dredge up troublesome memories, throwing the client back into the *fight or flight* crisis mode, shutting down their immune system.

There are *many* methods of eliminating stress and trauma. You've learned that it's possible to reduce, or even *permanently* eliminate stress and trauma in a variety of unusual ways.

The 6 techniques we've discussed—EFT, The Emotion Code, The Healing Code, Biophoton Therapy, Craniosacral Therapy and the Original Chi Machine—give us more oxygen, a better immune system and improved health. Most of them work with infants, people in comas and on animals. Some can be done yourself. Others you can do with a practitioner, in an office or, in some cases, long distance.

Some methods are more popular than others. For example, EFT has been used by millions of people but other methods are far less known. We saw how EFT tapping reversed multiple sclerosis in a disabled man,

*Final Thoughts*

allowing him to exit his wheelchair and start his own business.

We learned that it's possible, using The Emotion Code in a minute or two, to identify a problematic emotion that's trapped somewhere in the body, then *permanently* get rid of it using a refrigerator magnet. Eliminating a number of these negative emotions often leads to greater peace and less pain, stress and discomfort.

The Healing Code consists of saying some words and pointing fingers at special points on the face and neck. We saw how it eliminated *incurable* ALS for a doctor in less than 3 months.

We learned how 2 biophoton therapy sessions allowed a young lady to go several weeks without a seizure after experiencing seizures multiple times a week during her entire life.

Craniosacral Therapy is very good at releasing emotional problems and traumatic stress. We saw how it successfully corrected vertigo and treated trauma in an Olympic diver.

If we want additional oxygen, in minutes, you can get that with the Chi Machine. Just lie down and let the machine cause more oxygen to enter your bloodstream. It also allows corrective *chi* to flow throughout the body, often alleviating dozens of different pain and stress problems, as well as various illnesses.

## 6 LIFE CHANGING ENERGY HEALING METHODS

The methods in Part III of this book should help most people better deal with stressful and traumatic situations. My wife and I use a number of these methods regularly, as does my ten decades old mother. I invite you to try any of them if you're so inclined.

But if nothing changes in your life, your health and stress levels cannot improve. Neither of us wants that to happen. So, consider making one or more changes in your life. I hope you find something that reverses or reduces your pain, stress and illnesses.

Once again, I am *not* a doctor—so—it is your own responsibility to make sure that whatever you do is medically responsible. Consult with your doctors and medical professionals as needed and desired.

Blessings to you on your healing journey,

*John*

# Appendix A

# RESOURCES

## Books and CDs

***101 Miracles of Natural Healing* by** Luke Chan
***Alkalize or Die* by** Dr. Theodore A. Baroody
***Blink* by** Malcolm Gladwell
***Feelings Buried Alive Never Die ...* by** Karol Truman
***Flood Your Body with Oxygen* by** Ed McCabe
***Heal Your Body* by** Louise Hay
***Healing is Voltage* by** Jerry Tennant, MD
***Prayer is Good Medicine* by** Larry Dossey, MD
***Recovery From Parkinson's* by** Dr. Janice Walton-Hadlock, DAOM
***Secret Sounds* by** Jill Mattson
***Self-Healing with Sound and Music* CD by** Andrew Weil, MD and Kimba Arem
***The Biology of Belief* by** Bruce Lipton PhD
***The Brain's Way of Healing* by** Norman Doidge,

# 6 LIFE CHANGING ENERGY HEALING METHODS

MD

***The Collection*** by Nathan L. Lipton, MD (Chi Machine testimonials)

***The Emotion Code*** by Dr. Bradley Nelson

***The Genie in your Genes*** by Dawson Church, PhD

***The GenoType Diet*** by Dr. Peter J. Adamo with Catherine Whitney

***The Healing Code*** by Alexander Loyd, PhD, ND with Ben Johnson, MD, DO, NMD

***The Heart of Healing*** edited by Dawson Church

***The Power of Positive Thinking*** by Dr. Norman Vincent Peale

***The Relaxation Response*** by Herbert Benson, MD and Miriam Z. Klipper

***The Silva Mind Control Method*** by José Silva and Philip Miele

***The Stress of Life*** by Hans Selye, MD

***Think and Grow Rich*** by Napoleon Hill

***Your Inner Physician and You*** by Dr. John Upledger

***Vibrational Medicine*** by Richard Gerber, MD

# Websites

www.biontology.com (biophoton therapy website)
www.ChiChoices.com/chi-machine (Chi

Appendix A: Resources

Machine information)

**www.eftuniverse.com** (an informative EFT website)

**www.emofree.com/eft** (website of Gary Craig, founder of EFT)

**www.healerslibrary.com** (The Emotion Code and Body Code website)

**www.newmedicine.ca** (*German New Medicine* Website and ideas of Dr. Hamer)

**www.qnrt.com** (Quantum Neuro Reset Technique website)

**www.thehealingcodes.com** (The Healing Codes website)

**www.upledger.com** (Upledger Institute International craniosacral therapy information)

**www.upledger.org** (Upledger Foundation craniosacral therapy information)

## YouTube Videos (by title)

*Dr. Joseph Mercola speaks about EFT Tapping*

*Healing Code Demonstration final*

*Introduction to EFT, Gary Craig*

*The EFT Basic Recipe by Founder Gary Craig*

*Überraschend universelle Heilmethode—German (EFT video with German subtitles)*

## Other Videos (by title)

*Floor to Ceiling Eye Roll*

www.eftuniverse.com/video/eft-tapping-floor-to-ceiling-eye-roll-201

## How to find a practitioner

### EFT Practitioners

**www.eftuniverse.com/certified-eft-practitioners** (EFT Practitioners, most of whom can work by telephone)

**www.EFTprofessional.com** (EFT Practitioners, most of whom can work by telephone)

### The Emotion Code Practitioners

**www.healerslibrary.com/global-practitioner-map/** (Worldwide Emotion Code and Body Code practitioners)

**www.healerslibrary.com/services/** (Emotion Code and Body Code staff practitioners)

### The Healing Code Practitioners

**www.thehealingcodes.com/meet-practitioners** (Healing Codes practitioners, most of whom can work by telephone)

**Biophoton Therapy Practitioners**

**www.biontology.com/practitioners/find-a-practitioner** (Biophoton practitioners, called *biontologists*)

**Craniosacral Therapy Practitioners**

**www.iahp.com/pages/search/index.php** (Craniosacral therapists)

**The Original Chi Machine**

**www.chichoices.com/chi-machine** (Chi Machine information, including videos, how to use and how to purchase a machine to use *yourself* in your own home)

# More Resources for Readers

Information in this Resources Appendix, with clickable links, more current information, as well as with additional resource information, notes and comments, is available at:

**www.ChiChoices.com/energy-healing-resources**

My contact page (to avoid spam) is:

**www.ChiChoices.com/contact**

Please feel free to contact me, via the above contact page, if you have suggestions for this or another book or if you have any comments.

# Would You Do Me a Favor?

Thank you for reading this book which I hope you found enjoyable, informative, helpful and maybe even eye-opening.

Your *honest* review—which can be short—will help future readers discover how they might benefit from this book.

It can be left here, if you use Amazon USA:

www.amazon.com/dp/B01N9DXQF1

Here are Amazon's other English language sites where you can leave your review if your book was purchased outside the USA:

Canada   www.amazon.ca/dp/B01N9DXQF1

Ireland   www.amazon.co.uk/dp/B01N9DXQF1

U.K.   www.amazon.co.uk/dp/B01N9DXQF1

India   www.amazon.in/dp/B01N9DXQF1

Australia   www.amazon.com.au/d/B01N9DXQF1

If you scroll down to just below where reviews appear,

you'll see a button that says: "Write a customer review." You can click it to leave your review.

I read all reviews, appreciate them, and use them to learn how to better serve my readers.

Thank you for sharing your valuable time to write a brief review for me. It is *much* appreciated.

*John*

# For my Readers

## Additional Resources

Information in my *Resources Appendix*—and much more—is available here:

**www.ChiChoices.com/energy-healing-resources**

It has *clickable links* and contains *more resource* information than the *Resources Appendix*. In it you will find additional notes and explanatory comments about individual resources.

## Future Book Information

If you would like to know when my book is available in other formats or when my other planned books become available, you can join my readers list. You will *not* be deluged with email (which neither of us probably like). Just go to:

**www.ChiChoices.com/ourbooks**

# About the Author

Author John O'Dwyer became a *health nut* at age 27 and is now in his seventh decade. He loves people and enjoys reading health and other books, riding a bicycle, jogging, walking and doing tai chi.

He is a former nuclear submarine officer, mathematics teacher and computer programmer whose strength is making complicated things simple. His mission is to help pass on his extensive health knowledge to others in an engaging and informative way.

While he is *not* a doctor and makes *no* medical claims, the author does have certifications in several energy balancing methods. He has helped hundreds of people get free—or largely free—of pain and distress in minutes and has aided others over a longer period of time.

He enjoys learning foreign languages and spent 7 years abroad in Ireland, France, Japan and Canada either attending school, working or both. He has also lived in 11 different states and currently resides on the Mississippi Gulf Coast with his wife, Dorothy. They have 3 grown daughters.

Made in the USA
Middletown, DE
25 January 2018